# Mastering Microdosing

# Mastering Microdosing

*How to Use Sub-Perceptual
Psychedelics to Heal Trauma,
Improve Performance, and
Transform Your Life*

## Paul F. Austin

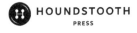

HOUNDSTOOTH
PRESS

**Mastering Microdosing**
*How to Use Sub-Perceptual Psychedelics to Heal Trauma,
Improve Performance, and Transform Your Life*

ISBN  978-1-5445-3508-1  Hardcover
       978-1-5445-3507-4  Paperback
       978-1-5445-3506-7  Ebook

# Contents

PART III

# What Microdosing Makes Possible

# PART I

# Why Microdosing

# 1

# Waves of Change

Microdosing may be a new concept for our modern world, but the intentional use of psychedelics goes back thousands of years. In fact, throughout human history, people have used psychedelic substances as tools to connect with the earth, with themselves, and with the divine. Early indigenous cultures centered much of their religious practices around various psychoactive plants native to wildly different environments.

In the deserts of Mexico, researchers carbon-dated ashes from a ceremonial fireplace used to burn the psychedelic peyote cactus at fifteen thousand years old. Gathering and consuming peyote is so emblematic of the Wixárika people that it is woven into their culture's origin story.[1]

In the Amazon jungle, ayahuasca has been used by curanderos, or shamans, for spiritual purposes for at least one thousand years.[2] The brew is made from the vine of one plant and the leaf of another: a combination arrived at with intention. When asked how they discovered the process of making ayahuasca, the curanderos often explain that the plants told their ancestors how to use them. Curanderos also keep a variety of other medicinal plants in their medicine bags meant to achieve altered states of consciousness, such as tobacco and yopo (a snuff with 5-MeO-DMT).

In the East, "the divine mushroom of immortality" known as soma is described in several iconic, ancient Indian texts, including the Vedas, the Bhagavad Gita, and the Upanishads.[3] Soma was said to produce intense sensations of bliss, poetic inspiration, and an expanded awareness of reality. Scholars debate what substances were the basis for soma; some theorize soma is the *psilocybe cubensis* mushroom, while others think it may have been a combination of cannabis and ephedrine. What we know for certain is that it was a psychoactive substance taken in a ceremonial context to expand consciousness.

The diversity of these three examples—a cactus from North America, a vine from the Amazon, and a mushroom from India— illustrates our deep, human desire to seek a connection between ourselves and the spiritual plane.

In the West, our long tradition with psychedelics began in Greece. There, ancient inscriptions from religious temples describe the importance of psychedelic sacraments: "Life would not be worth living without *kykeon*."[4]

Kykeon was a psychedelic drink made from ergot, a fungus

that grows on rye. If the name of this psychedelic is unfamiliar, its modern counterpart is likely not: ergot is the base ingredient that, after several chemical reactions, becomes LSD.

The journey ergot has taken through time, from kykeon to LSD, mirrors the use of psychedelic sacraments across the span of Western history. One truth I often come back to is the cyclical nature of time: history isn't linear, and it continues to repeat itself. Our Western lineage with psychedelics is no exception.

There have been three distinct periods when we've utilized psychedelics as integral tools for healing, transcendence, and transformation. I call these periods "waves." The First Wave orients around the ancient use of these sacraments. The Second Wave came about with the countercultural movement in the 1950s and '60s. The Third Wave, as I will detail later, is now.

## The First Wave

In ancient Greece, kykeon was likely only available in private circles of elite society. Every year, people gathered in Eleusis, a town about twenty miles outside of Athens, to engage in secret ritualistic ceremonies known as the Eleusinian Mysteries. There, participants drank kykeon as a psychedelic sacrament. Both Plato and Aristotle credit the Eleusinian Mysteries as a turning point for their understanding of reality, which means that much of the foundation of Western philosophy emerged from psychedelic-induced experiences.[5]

Knowing this, you could say that psychedelics are responsible for, or at least etched into, the foundation of Western philosophy. The Eleusinian Mysteries provide both an example and a comparison of how we have historically used psychedelics and how we can better leverage them today.

The ancient Greeks engaged in a tried-and-true practice for catalyzing ego death by drinking kykeon. The Eleusinian Mysteries revolved around the cult of Dionysus, the Greek god of wine and psychoactives, among other things. By having male and female characteristics, he embodied the paradox of divinity. He was also the "dying and rising" god, transforming his followers through an initiation of death and rebirth.

So, the Greeks drank kykeon—likely in large quantities—to have reality-altering experiences that allowed them to lose all sense of self. An ancient Greek inscription describes the importance of this ritual for managing the inevitable fear of death that every human shares: "If you die before you die, you will not die when you die."[6]

While many other tools initiate mystical experiences—meditation, fasting, flagellation, and extreme sensory deprivation, to name a few—none are as reliable as the psychedelic experience. And that's not just my opinion; recent research confirms that psychedelic substances, when used within an intentional container, consistently and reliably induce a mystical experience.[7]

When the Roman Empire made Christianity its official religion, they prohibited psychedelic sacraments, thus ending the

First Wave. Psychedelics wouldn't come back on the scene—at least, not in a significant way—until the 1950s, during what we colloquially refer to as the Second Wave.

Even so, it is only in relatively recent times, since the days of Descartes, Frances Bacon, and the onset of scientism and materialist reductionism in the fifteenth and sixteenth centuries, that Western culture has fully stigmatized mystical experiences and placed nearly all its confidence in the linear, rational world of science and the scientific method.

While advancements in science and technology have brought tremendous abundance to twenty-first-century life, they have also led to a sweeping, dramatic disconnection from our essence—an alienation from the Oneness described for eons by philosophers and mystics. Some call this sense of connection our true nature; others know it as the Godhead. Whatever we name it, the consequences of disconnecting from the "Source" are many: rising rates of anxiety and depression, the blind destruction of our environment, and an inescapable sense of all meaning being lost from life.

We've reached a ceiling in our drive toward money and status, and we're looking for new, inspired perspectives—particularly around ways to reconnect to Oneness, Source, the ineffable.

## The Second Wave

The Second Wave of psychedelics, more commonly known as the "counterculture," launched the first pushback against an ultra-conformist society devoid of mystery, awe, and reverence. Two events catalyzed the second wave: Albert Hofmann's discovery of LSD's psychedelic properties in 1943 and Robert Gordon Wasson's experiences with the "magic mushroom" in Oaxaca, Mexico, in the 1950s.

In 1957, Wasson published his experience in *Life Magazine* with a photo essay entitled "Seeking the Magic Mushroom." With the publication of this article, the counterculture of psychedelics took off.

As Wasson's *Life* article woke up the public, researchers were actively studying the benefits and risks of psychedelic medicine. In the '50s and '60s, over one thousand clinical papers were published on the efficacy of LSD for everything from alcoholism to anxiety, to depression, to addiction, to OCD, and to autism. There was a substantial amount of clinical evidence amassed about the potential of LSD as an aid for mental health. Researchers also developed a phenomenal framework around psychedelic-assisted psychotherapy, which garnered interest and attention from scientists, healers, and the broader public. This increased interest, awareness, and use of psychedelics had ripple effects for increasing our sense of interconnectedness in modern culture.

For example, the movement around ecological awareness may have looked entirely different if not for psychedelics. In 1966, Stewart Brand (who is still alive at the time of writing) had an LSD trip supervised by Dr. James Fadiman (also still alive). At that point, Fadiman was an up-and-coming psychologist exploring the intersection of psychedelics and creativity.

During his experience, Stewart realized that NASA had yet to release satellite images of Earth from space. He believed that seeing photos of the whole earth would change the way people thought about and treated Mother Nature. He petitioned the federal government to release a photo of the earth from space, and he secured hundreds of thousands of signatures for the petition. After several years of foot-dragging, the government finally released a photo. That image impacted society so powerfully, that it inspired the first Earth Day. This became an annual celebration that continues to bring awareness to the importance of caring for our ecosystems.

Similarly, the use of LSD in Palo Alto at Stanford University inspired the computer revolution. When early computer pioneers came out of their LSD experiences, they wanted to create technology that could better enable connection and communication between people. Two of the most resonant examples of this are:

1. Douglas Engelbart, who invented both the computer interface and the computer mouse, talked about how LSD influenced his work.
2. Steve Jobs, founder of Apple, claimed LSD use as one of the three most important, impactful, and profound experiences of his life.

Further, the increasing consumption of psychedelics amplified the myriad movements for civil rights, ecological rights, and pacifist rights in the US. Invigorated by a sense of interconnect-edness intrinsic to psychedelics, people came together to march, protest, and participate in grassroots movements while demanding change.

This became a central problem for the Nixon administration. Former Nixon Domestic Policy Chief John Ehrlichman later described the situation to *Harper's Magazine* writer, Dan Baum:

> The Nixon campaign in 1968 and the Nixon White House after that had two enemies: the antiwar left and Black people. You understand what I'm saying? We knew we couldn't make it illegal to be either against the war or Black, but by getting the public to associate the hippies with marijuana as well as LSD and Blacks with heroin, and then criminalizing both heavily, we could disrupt those communities. We could arrest their leaders, raid their homes, break up their meetings and vilify them night after night on the evening news. Did we know we were lying about the drugs? Of course we did.[8]

Richard Nixon began waging the "War on Drugs" in 1971, with the explicit goal of destabilizing the hippie left. This brought the Second Wave of psychedelics to an abrupt halt. By putting the lid on psychedelic use, the military-industrial complex was able to continue integrating its destructive principles and values into the mainstream, most noticeably its "grow at all costs" mindset.

We were taught that if GDP isn't growing, then something is wrong. And yet, we live on a planet with finite resources. If we don't learn to use these resources sustainably, we'll end up like all formerly extinct ancient civilizations: a blip of consciousness in time, never to be seen or heard from again.

We're currently experiencing a hangover from living under these destructive principles for the past fifty years. One of these Nixon-era principles defined which drugs are legal and acceptable to consume—alcohol, tobacco, and coffee—and which drugs are illegal and considered harmful to consume. This framing led to the rise of private prisons and created a financial incentive to incarcerate users of the "bad" drugs. It also led to a fifty-year hiatus on psychedelic research, one of the most destructive aspects of this policy.

Thankfully, the US government couldn't keep the lid on psychedelics forever. Eventually, the genie began to find its way back out of the bottle.

## The Third Wave

Today, we are witnessing a looming ecological crisis, peak work dissatisfaction, and all-time high levels of addiction, suicide, and PTSD. Clearly, something is wrong.[9]

As people begin rediscovering and experimenting with psychedelics, it has become increasingly clear that the Nixon era War on Drugs was a misinformation campaign that held society—and personal healing—back. With a plethora of information available through the internet, more people are "waking up" and recognizing how imbalanced Western society has become. Though times are changing, Nixon's harmful drug policies still dominate the political landscape today. For example, LSD is still federally classified as a Schedule 1 drug. As of the publication of this book, so is cannabis (despite its legalization in several states).

Now, more than ever, people are aware that not all leaders have the public's best interests at heart. It's no coincidence that more people today are taking ownership of their well-being, rather than trusting society to care for them. Whether the trends are conscious or subconscious, people are increasingly turning to activities such as yoga, mindfulness meditation, hiking, vegetarianism or veganism, and functional fitness based on evolutionary principles. We must recognize that it's up to us as individuals to facilitate healing and transformation. And, to succeed on that journey, we can't underestimate the importance of optimizing our physical, emotional, and spiritual health.

Psychedelics are an excellent tool for optimal healing. Unfortunately, because the psychedelic experience brings awareness to principles that oppose the "grow at all costs" mindset, they have been demonized by the US government (and, as a result, most modern nation-state governments). The government's inaccurate portrayal of the psychedelic experience has left the public badly misinformed and has created a nearly insurmountable cultural stigma around the use of psychedelics.

Fortunately, the cultural conversation around psychedelics has changed once again, thanks to three core factors:

1. Research on the efficacy of psychedelics as medicine
2. Well-known individuals "coming out" in support of such substances
3. Shifting dialogue around previous illicit substances like cannabis

For instance, Michael Pollan's book about the science of psychedelics, *How to Change Your Mind*, was a number one *New York Times* bestseller in 2018. At the time of writing *Mastering Microdosing*, hundreds of millions of dollars have been invested into researching the use of psychedelic substances for mental health care, and hundreds of companies have popped up to participate. The media response and coverage have been incredibly positive overall. Now, many people see psychedelics as powerful tools that can help address the mental health, ecological, and spiritual crises we currently face.

Laws are changing, too. Oregon legalized psilocybin, making it legally available for therapeutic use in 2023. Detroit, Seattle, and Oakland have decriminalized all plant medicines. This is a massive breakthrough for the Third Wave psychedelic movement, whose members were (and still are in some areas) imprisoned for exploring the realms of inner consciousness.

Psychedelics can provide people with tremendously powerful, transformative experiences. Of course, not everyone is seeking a complete ego death and subsequent rebirth. That's why the Third Wave of psychedelics is built upon a unique approach: microdosing.

Microdosing involves taking very small doses of a substance—in this case, psychedelics—in order to benefit without experiencing powerful hallucinogenic effects. So, while the world slowly begins to reopen itself to psychedelics, microdosing offers assistance that can reach and help more people more quickly.

Microdosing supplements are now sold publicly in Vancouver, Venice Beach, and even Vermont. The microdosing subreddit has grown from 20,000 to 220,000-plus people over the past few years. The result of this cultural exposure is that a formerly "bad" drug is being rediscovered for its many positive properties, especially when taken in a small dose.

Even someone like my dad, whose boomer generation saw the vilification of LSD in the media during the War on Drugs, has gotten over his skepticism and has embraced microdosing. As a young man, news reports inundated him with stories that equated the LSD experience to a psychotic break—something that would leave a person "never the same again." Like others of his generation, he was reasonably afraid to take a large dose all at once. However, he was willing to dabble in a microdose that allowed him to experience some of the tangible benefits without losing absolute and total control over his psyche and consciousness.

By choosing to be open to experimentation, the older generation is experiencing something extraordinary. They're noting that microdosing gives them energy, improves cognitive function, and sparks a long-lost sense of vitality full of the beauty and joy that tends to dissipate as one grows older. It helps them to remain curious and open, rather than stuck in their ways. In a way, micro-dosing helps them stay connected to the awe of life.

What's more, microdosing allows people to shift their life experience without a total and complete system shock. This approach makes intuitive sense when explored through the lens of a swimming metaphor. When we learned to swim as children, we started in the shallow end with a swimming instructor. This enabled us to learn how to be in the water without risking the potential trauma of drowning. Bit by bit, as our skills and comfort grew, we branched out into deeper water, free of any and all constraints. Similarly, by experimenting with microdosing, individuals learn to swim in the shallow end of their consciousness before diving into a high dose.

Microdosing allows people to experience a slightly altered state of consciousness, calming their fears and allowing them to become familiar with the profound benefits of psychedelics. If someone only reads about the experience of "dying before you die," they're less likely take the initial high dose plunge. However, someone who takes the first step through microdosing is much more likely to do a high dose later.

### What, Exactly, Is Microdosing?

Microdosing, by definition, involves consuming sub-perceptual doses of psychedelics—most commonly LSD and psilocybin—in a set protocol, typically two to three times per week for one to two months.

Unlike "macrodosing," microdosing is not a "special occasion" event. Instead, it integrates psychedelic consumption into your daily routine to boost creativity, improve energy and health, increase mental focus, and help you better connect with others. Especially alongside a mindfulness practice such as meditation or yoga, a microdosing protocol can have profound benefits for well-being and productivity.

Microdosing is used to effectively treat mild to severe mental health issues. This practice has also helped people whose symptoms were not severe enough to warrant pharmaceutical intervention get their mental health back to baseline. Those who have suffered from clinical depression for many years and have potentially cycled through many pharmaceuticals find that microdosing can help them get off their medications.

Microdosing can also help people with traumatic brain injuries activate new connections in the brain, enabling greater functionality on a day-to-day basis. Microdosing has helped people with PTSD by allowing them to process the root of their trauma and to integrate it so that it no longer unconsciously directs their life.

At Third Wave, the psychedelic platform I started in 2015, we have seen ample evidence that the attention given to microdosing will be a driving force for integrating psychedelics within mainstream society. Already, we have seen examples of scientific research impacting public policy with decriminalization efforts. The FDA has also granted breakthrough approval status to MDMA-assisted psychotherapy for PTSD and to psilocybin for treatment-resistant depression and major depressive disorder. These substances have been fast-tracked for approval because the clinical efficacy is so strong.

As research continues, and as prominent individuals "come out of the psychedelic closet," the stigma around these powerful substances will recede. More people will become properly educated about how to utilize psychedelics in an intentional, structured way. Some examples of celebrities who have spoken openly about their psychedelic experiences include Will Smith in his new autobiography, *Will*: "This was my first tiny taste of freedom," Smith writes of his first experience on ayahuasca. "In my fifty-plus years on this planet, this is the unparalleled greatest feeling I've ever had."[10]

Brad Pitt has talked to the *New York Times* about why microdosing has been so helpful for him.[11] The list of celebrities who have been impacted by psychedelics is constantly growing: Miley Cyrus, Megan Fox, and Machine Gun Kelly have all spoken highly of ayahuasca; Mike Tyson has spoken about his experiences with 5-MeO-DMT; former NBA star Lamar Odom has spoken about ketamine. A Netflix series called "Have a Good Trip" features celebrities talking about their psychedelic experiences, including ASAP Rocky, Carrie Fisher, Anthony Bourdain, Adam Levine, Deepak Chopra, Ben Stiller, and many more. Each time someone well-known speaks publicly about their psychedelic use, the movement gains a bit of traction.

I won't pretend that spreading the word will be easy or that everyone will get the message right away, no matter how strong the science or the number of celebrity endorsements. However, tangible change is happening all around us. Even between this book's first and second editions, the culture around psychedelics has vastly changed. It's much better received than a few years ago, largely thanks to positive media coverage and additional research. When I published the first edition in 2018, psychedelic research was still considered fringe, but now it is popular—even sexy.

So, where does microdosing fall into this still-evolving history?

By spreading the word on microdosing, we are cultivating awareness about a new era of psychedelic use. In this Third Wave, we will educate individuals on the responsible and measured use of psychedelic substances for specific purposes. We won't make the same mistakes people made in the First—and particularly the Second—Wave. Unlike the counterculture movement of the '60s and '70s, when people used psychedelics to reject mainstream values, microdosing will imbue mainstream society with the values of the psychedelic experience without requiring a complete and total disconnect.

Now, instead of encouraging pushback against mainstream narratives—and thus setting ourselves up to be perceived as the "other"—the Third Wave of psychedelics promotes the integration of these powerful substances to construct new models in society.

These new models will recognize the interconnectedness of all things and help people turn away from the mindless materialism and consumerism that has destroyed the ecological capital on which we rely.

In other words, the Second Wave encouraged separation; the Third Wave encourages integration and the act of coming together.

In that spirit, it seems only fair that we continue with my own story, as the story of my life may resonate with your own experience and your interest in microdosing.

## Three Failures and a Revelation

My story is typical of our times. Born and raised in a traditional Midwestern, suburban home, I grew up in a family and community that espoused the pillar values of Christianity: humility, kindness, support, and love.

My parents went the extra mile to provide me with every suburban American opportunity: private violin lessons, excellent public schools, church every Sunday, and competitive, elite sports.

My early years were not, however, carefree. Growing up in a profoundly Calvinist culture, I was bombarded with warnings against all sorts of potential transgressions.

Drugs? Bad.

Sex? Bad.

Thinking different? *Real bad.*

Like many kids, I went along with this belief system during childhood and my early teens. Then, one day, the unavoidable occurred: my youthful discontent and rebellion intersected with receiving my driver's license, meaning I was free to roam and do as I pleased. My best friend at the time was an atheist—an anomaly amidst our religious community. I looked up to him for his ability to think and act independently, which complemented our natural teenage pull toward rebellion. This friend introduced me to cannabis.

The idea of teenagers introducing each other to illicit drugs may seem like a stereotype. However, as I look back on this time in my life, there was no "dangerous path" I walked. I was sixteen and safe in the confines of a concrete hippie hut with my three friends when I smoked my first blunt. It was the first time I ever consumed a psychoactive substance.

Using cannabis encouraged me to individuate and think critically. Imbibing such a sacred plant inspired me to challenge the culture I'd been raised in. Finally, I began to discover and defend my own beliefs.

While much of my community regarded cannabis consumption as a sure sign of failure, I remember the experience as mostly positive. Despite the undercurrents of paranoia that came with doing something illegal, I enjoyed the giggling and the general sense of euphoria I experienced while under the influence of this supposedly "bad, life-destroying drug." It seemed that everything my elders had told me about it was wrong. Naturally, I started wondering what else they were wrong about.

Over the next couple months, I kept experimenting. I tried cannabis two more times before the inevitable happened: my parents found out.

My parents felt they knew what was "best" for me and grounded me for a month. After all, the United States government had "properly educated" them about the dangers and harms of mari-juana. The logic went like this: it was illegal because it was bad—and it was bad because it was illegal. Plus, everyone knew that smoking weed led to stupidity and laziness and eventually to a miserable life of hard drugs and poverty.

I was not convinced.

I didn't learn to avoid drugs as my parents had hoped. Like many suburban American teenagers, I simply kept my family life and social life separate instead. Regardless of the generation in which you grew up, you likely learned similar lessons.

My next "societal failure" came at the age of nineteen, when I took LSD for the first time. While the reaction of my community was a deep disappointment—"How could you!"—I registered a different message. I finally came alive to the wondrous awe of life, love, and nature. For the first time, I saw through the veil of superficial modernity and dove deep into what really matters in life: relationships, community, and love.

Until that moment, I had accepted the deep disconnection of modern life as just the way things were. Humans are social animals. When we live alongside everyone else going about their daily business in the modernized, industrialized world, we think the overt disconnection is normal. I certainly did. Then LSD catalyzed a profound shift in my life, and, as cliché as it sounds, I was never the same again.

This change manifested in two distinct ways. The first was retrospective healing. I'd grown up in a community that greatly emphasized conformity, shaming anyone who was an independent thinker. On my first acid trip, I realized that the shame and guilt were external and did not belong to me. I didn't have to continue to live that story. That realization was incredibly healing, and afterward, I stopped being so hard on myself for the expectations imposed upon me by society.

The second way LSD changed me was by removing the fear of death. That Greek inscription that references death-before-death is accurate. I experienced ego dissolution and was able to see through the veil to the other side, which led me to realize that death is an illusion.

So many of our actions are dictated by the fear—both conscious and unconscious—of death. But once that fear is removed, the choices we make come from a place of freedom and liberation and, therefore, are much more honest and authentic. After LSD, I became inspired to pursue a more unconventional life path, embracing radical responsibility in every choice. The more responsibility I took for the direction of my life, the more fulfilling and meaningful it became. I opted not to be driven or incentivized by external motivators. Steadied by my internal callings and desires, I stopped chasing money, status, and other conventional ego-boosters.

My third point of "failure" came at the age of twenty. As a university sophomore, I wanted to make some extra cash. Having already exhausted my work options, I chose to sell cannabis on the side. It was a small operation. I primarily sold baggies to friends who lived nearby. I lived in a bubble of White privilege provided by the liberal arts university I attended. Of course, what I was doing was still illegal and therefore dangerous.

I sold weed to White college students for about nine months without the slightest repercussion. However, the one Hispanic kid I sold to was trailed by the cops, a move which exemplifies the racial motivations behind the War on Drugs.

They pulled him over, found the weed, and he gave me up.

I was so naïve when the cops showed up at my house that I didn't even ask if they had a warrant. I just let them into my home and told them everything. They said if I cooperated, they wouldn't arrest me. I gave them the small amount of weed I had left, the $7,000 cash in my safe, and the name of someone else who was selling weed.

Because I gave someone else up, I didn't get arrested. I never got fingerprinted, handcuffed, or interrogated, and I never heard from the police again. Though I'd suffered no harsh repercussions, I was still traumatized.

It took me a year to get over this encounter with the law. In processing this experience, I became so enraged at the system that I took matters into my own hands, doing everything possible to help overturn the ridiculous War on Drugs. Getting "busted" awoke a deep-seated anger, one that inspired my initial foray into shifting the public's perception of psychedelic medicines. From this experience, I made an internal commitment to change the system in which we currently live.

I made this vow because I knew I wasn't alone in my numerous failures to adapt to a sick and broken world. Countless others who have grown up in our industrialized Western world have experienced something similar. As Jiddu Krishnamurti said, "It is no measure of health to be well adjusted to a profoundly sick society."

Now, more than ten years after that initial bust, psychedelics are at the precipice of mainstream acceptance. They are increasingly understood as medicines and not just playthings of high school dropouts and hippies. Psychedelics, more than almost any other cutting-edge substance, provide hope for a more humane, compassionate, and interconnected world.

Using psychedelics helped me understand that I could pursue a life of fulfillment and entrepreneurship without hopping onto the hedonic treadmill of arbitrary life milestones. Once I'd glimpsed the truth, I knew I could never conform.

Absolute failure happens when we adjust and adapt to a culture built on consumerism, individualism, and the destruction of ecological capital. In other words, my biggest failure was my inability to conform to the poisonous values and principles of modern society, including dogmatic religion, rampant consumerism, and normative drug use. I refused to buy into the soul-sucking cycle of modern adulthood: incurring debt for things that the culture says you need, like an expensive car, a college education, and a big house, until you're trapped in a terrible job that you hate, just so you can afford all the shit you don't actually need.

If I hadn't lived through these "failures," I never would have written a book on a taboo topic like psychedelics. Had I chosen to pursue a more conventional lifestyle and jumped into the rat race like most people in their twenties, thirties, and forties, it would be nearly impossible for me to step out of the shadows and expose myself as a psychedelic "user."

Psychedelics wake you up to the truth of who you are. In that awakening, you have a choice: burn the ships and go courageously into the unknown, or live a conventional life of meekness, walking along the path that's been established without genuinely listening to what your soul wants.

## Rebellion Turns to Productivity

One reason I can speak out publicly about the importance of psychedelic substances is that I had a fortunate—if not conventional—upbringing in many ways.

While misguided in their attempts to protect me from the world of illicit drugs, my parents provided a stable home. I grew up in a house overflowing with love, care, and compassion. I also enjoyed some practical benefits of landing in this family and community. As the son of a university administrator, I received a free college education, leaving me with no student debt—a rare privilege for an American university student today. Because of my freedom from debt, I could pursue work with less attachment to financial remuneration and more focus on pursuing my passions.

What I yearned for was exotic—I sought experiences that, stripped of comfort and convenience, would place me far outside my usual "comfort zone," requiring significant adaptation to a new way of living. So, upon graduating from university, I moved to Turkey, where I taught English for a year.

My spirit of unconventionality continued to burn, growing with every passing day, consuming untold amounts of time and energy. I immersed myself in a comprehensive self-study of all things entrepreneurial. From these many hours of rigorous research grew my first online business—TOEFL Speaking Teacher (TST)—a niche online English school focused on preparing international students for a problematic English entrance exam through one-to-one and group coaching.

My North Star is freedom—to express, to create, and to be—and I began to understand that to create true freedom in my life, I would have to be an entrepreneur. I saw entrepreneurship as a path toward cultivating greater freedom for my soul. Sure, there are finances involved in entrepreneurship. But financial remuneration has never been my North Star.

In fact, it was quite the opposite. I was drawn to entrepreneurship because it's something you can't bullshit. If you don't create value, you'll quickly end up broke and back at square one. You get immediate feedback about what's working and what's not.

I set myself up with a full-time job teaching English that covered my financial necessities. I lived nomadically, moving to Thailand, then Portugal, then Budapest. I was in a place of freedom that, should a diamond opportunity arise, I would be able to take it. And when three friends and I got the idea for Third Wave, that's precisely what I did.

## The Way Forward

In July 2015, two friends visited me while I lived in Budapest. Both had previous experience with psychedelics and were interested in the surging trend of microdosing. We began our time together with a microdose of LSD and a thorough exploration of the magnificent city of Budapest. After an excellent first experience, we chose to step up our game and consume 250 micrograms of acid in the city's foothills two days later.

We awoke at 6:30 a.m. and each took a couple of tabs of acid. Then we called an Uber to drive us to Normafa, Budapest's largest park, overlooking the Danube and the area's cascading hills. LSD typically takes forty-five minutes to kick in, and so, just as we began "peaking," we settled into a beautiful meadow with spectacular views of the city.

My friend had a profound experience because this was the first time he'd done acid in twenty years. His primary reaction was, "What have I been missing this whole time?" He felt revitalized, sharp, and incredibly alive. So did I. Our conversation kept returning to the question, "Why don't more people know about this?" We discussed the high likelihood that psychedelics would follow cannabis's trajectory from an illicit substance to a widely accepted and legal one.

One big issue we saw with the public's ability to embrace psychedelics was the lack of information available in the mainstream media. Tim Ferriss, for his part, had become an outspoken advocate of psychedelics on his blog and podcast. Aside from that, most of the information out there came in the form of some random Geocities website, which no rational person would ever consider a viable source. There was nothing out there that would reach the average person.

This is how we arrived at the idea to build a website that presents psychedelic education in a readily available form for the public. I'd be able to combine my love of teaching, my love of history, and my passion for psychedelics. This was what my soul craved.

While living in Budapest, I frequented a cafe serving "third wave coffee." That's where we got the name idea—the Third Wave of Psychedelics resonated immediately because we knew we were at its cusp. Humans were about to dive into psychedelic use for the third time in history, and microdosing would characterize this renaissance.

Over the next several days, we wrote out the Third Wave philosophy, based on three profound realizations we had during our trip.

- **Realization #1:** *The future of psychedelic use would be less about "getting high" and more about harnessing its tangible benefits in everyday life: vitality, connection, and creativity.* Psychedelics are valuable tools with practical benefits.

We knew we could give others the education they needed to use these tools wisely.

- **Realization #2:** *Psychedelics had a PR problem, and we wanted to fix it.* With the growing body of research in psychedelics and the reevaluation of cannabis's status as an illicit substance, we knew that more and more people would be interested in using psychedelic substances for personal benefit and growth. However, we also recognized that to make this really "catch on," the "hippie" vibe of the '60s needed to be stripped away and replaced by an aesthetic and brand that modern, mainstream culture could identify with.

- **Realization #3:** *Science and influencers can work together to spread the message.* As clinical research into psychedelics continues to grow, influencers can play an essential role by amplifying all the scientific progress.

It was time for the Third Wave to hit, but why? What had changed since the Second Wave crested? And why was *this* the right cultural moment for microdosing to take hold?

## Microdosing versus Pharmaceuticals

As a modality, psychedelics are much more efficacious than other drugs that people attempt to weave into their daily lives. Most people who microdose do so to improve their performance, so let's look at microdosing compared to performance-enhancing drugs such as Ritalin, Adderall, and Modafinil, as well as SSRIs such as Zoloft and Prozac.

Microdosing, proponents report, brings equal or better mental benefits than these pharmaceuticals, but in a gentler and healthier way. In an article for *WIRED*, pharmacology professor and psychedelic researcher Dr. David Nichols hypothesized that microdosing works as a stimulant by activating dopamine pathways and exciting the central cortex, like the effects of Adderall and Ritalin but without addictive properties or other harmful side effects.[12]

In this comparison, the first thing to note is that psychedelics are not addictive. There is no physiological dependence on these substances, so if you wish to stop using them, it is effortless to do so. This is a major contributing factor to their popularity.

Furthermore, when people use microdosing instead of using Adderall or the other amphetamines for performance enhancement, they report being much more playful and less rigid, while still maintaining focus and flow. The focus is not overwhelming, so users enjoy what they're doing.

People discover that through microdosing, they can bring more passion and playfulness to the work they're doing, and they can do the same amount of work in a shorter amount of time because they're able to access a flow state more frequently.

Next, let's compare psychedelics to SSRI medications like Zoloft and Prozac. Many people find that though their pharmaceutical medications were initially effective, sometime down the line, the efficacy wanes. They also find that though they manage their symptoms of depression or PTSD, these feelings are handled at the expense of feeling other emotions. Some people on SSRIs report feeling numb, deadened, or profoundly bored with the experience of living. Of course, that's better than feeling suicidal. But if there is a way to manage the symptoms of depression and PTSD while still feeling liveliness, joy, connection, and love—well, that's better all around.

As a result, people are looking to microdosing to help wean off pharmaceuticals. Instead of merely managing symptoms, psychedelics help people handle the root cause of those symptoms. Especially at higher doses, psychedelics make it very clear what matters to us, what is essential, and why we do what we do. Once we have a chance to heal the trauma of our past, we have more space for expansion, freedom, and self-expression.

Collectively, we are waking up to the knowledge that we can have complete alignment between all areas and aspects of our lives. We can have a job we like *and* that pays us well. We can have a stable partnership that's *also* healthy, nourishing, and intimate. We don't have to lose to gain, and microdosing with intention and awareness brings us closer to that understanding.

## Building the Future

The intention and awareness packed into microdosing has permanently and positively impacted my life. Through my own experiences, both in working with psychedelics and in speaking with others whose lives were transformed from microdosing, I came to believe in the promise of microdosing.

However, when I was first embarking on this venture, I still had a few lingering questions:

- How do we create a message about psychedelics that resonates with a mainstream crowd and shows psychedelics as something "normal" folks do?
- How do we start building bridges with the most influential people in society, with an understanding that psychedelics and particularly microdosing can help us build a better world?
- Why has microdosing—an area of psychedelics without a long history of clinical research—taken off in popularity at this particular time?

By exploring these questions, I realized that we stand in a unique spot today. We have arrived at a place where microdosing psychedelics for enhanced well-being, accelerated skill development, and expanded self-awareness is ready to go mainstream. What better avenue to mainstreaming psychedelics, I thought, than curating an informed, palatable, and nonthreatening message about their benefits? And who better to do it than the leaders who will build the future in which we'll live?

Consider the impact of the invention of the printing press:

before the printing press, those who could read and write were primarily priests and other religious figures—therefore, they were the ones who had control over the flow and dissemination of information. But with the invention of the printing press, literacy was democratized. Once 10 percent of the population became literate, these individuals built the necessary systems to bring about the Age of Enlightenment.

Everyone didn't have to become literate all at once to create systemic change. And today, similarly, not everyone—or even the majority—must embrace psychedelics for the movement to be potent. Ten percent can inspire massive change. We call this a Power Law, or the Law of Ten.

What I got from microdosing—presence, engagement, intimacy, flow states, leadership development, and more—transcended my initial desires. What I thought would be a nice little hack to overcome procrastination became a practice that completely transformed my approach to work, relationships, and, generally, life.

And now, I want to share why this beneficial practice may also transform yours.

## Want to Go Deeper?

Check out your *Microdosing Mastery* portal for exclusive resources, articles, and interviews to discover more about the topics from this chapter.

Just go to thethirdwave.co/bonus to access your exclusive book bonuses.

# 2

# The Microdosing Experience

Microdosing is having a moment. The basic concept of microdosing, however, is nothing new. Indeed, various indigenous groups have taken microdoses of psychedelic plants for hundreds, even thousands, of years. Terence McKenna went so far as to credit massive leaps in our evolutionary path to *Homo erectus*' consumption of psilocybin mushrooms during pack hunting.[13]

More recently, Albert Hofmann, who first synthesized LSD in 1938, considered microdosing one of the drug's most promising and least researched applications. He was among the first to experience its antidepressant and cognition-enhancing potential,[14] famously taking between 10 and 20 μg (micrograms) twice a week, for the last few decades of his life.[15]

Before becoming a proponent of microdosing, Hofmann was the first person to ever trip on LSD. In 1943, curious about the effects of the chemical he'd synthesized, Hofmann took 250 micrograms, thinking it was a small amount. This dosage was more than ten times the microdoses he would take in his later life.

He ended up tripping his face off while riding his bike home from the office in a nightmarish hallucination, imagining himself chased by demons. Once home, his wife cared for him through the end of the trip. Later, Hofmann described the trip to be immensely beneficial despite the terror he experienced. Because of this clear and tangible impact, he encouraged his pharmaceutical company, Sandoz, to give away as much LSD as possible to research institutions. That way, it could be tested for potential medicinal properties within psychiatric spheres.

When Robert Gordon Wasson published his 1957 *Life Magazine* article, "Seeking the Magic Mushroom," he caught the attention of two Harvard faculty members, Timothy Leary and Richard Alpert, who decided they'd go to Mexico to try magic mushrooms out for themselves. Their experience was so incredible that they decided to continue studying these mushrooms on their return to Harvard.

They ran into difficulties sourcing psilocybin at Harvard but discovered that, thanks to Sandoz's efforts to promote research, it was very easy to get LSD. So, Leary and Alpert started doing experimental research with LSD, using their Harvard graduate students as test subjects. Their research methods drew scrutiny from the school's administration, and Leary and Alpert were fired in 1963.

Thankfully, their dismissal from Harvard didn't have much of a detrimental effect on psychedelic research. By this time, research was happening all over the country. Stanford University was a leader in the field, and one person who got involved with the program was Ken Kesey, author of *One Flew Over the Cuckoo's Nest*. His psychedelic experiences so moved him that he went on to form The Merry Pranksters, a group of artists whose experiments with psychedelics resulted in chaotic, wonderfully exciting artwork. Some of the most famous members of The Merry Pranksters were members of a band called The Warlocks, who would later be known as The Grateful Dead.

The wild, counterculture lifestyle of The Merry Pranksters was cataloged in culture critic Tom Wolfe's *The Electric Kool-Aid Acid Tests*. He detailed how, during The Merry Pranksters' infamous "Acid Tests," a sizable group of people would take LSD in an effort to transcend reality and connect to a higher plane. Unfortunately, Wolfe's descriptions of the nonconformist group's escapades contributed to the subsequent crackdown against the widespread use of LSD.

With the explosion of psychedelics happening coast to coast, there was too much chaos for the culture to handle. This all came to a head in 1966, known as "The Summer of Love." So many people were taking high doses of acid in San Francisco that the governor of California made LSD illegal. Soon enough, the federal government followed suit, making LSD illegal throughout the United States.

The future of LSD research would have to shift to differentiate itself from the rapidly growing cultural stigma around psychedelics.

## From Macro to Micro

In the early-2000s, upon learning about Albert Hofmann's microdosing protocol, psychedelic researcher Dr. James Fadiman set his sights on studying microdosing. He'd already studied the creativity- and concentration-boosting effects of LSD and mescaline (at moderate doses) during the 1960s. In 2008, he put together a self-study protocol with clinical psychologist Dr. Sophia Korb, and began soliciting reports from users, hoping to map out this uncharted area of a psychedelic experience.

I was fortunate to speak with Dr. Fadiman on the Third Wave podcast. In the interview, we dove into his early LSD experiments, namely, a study he published in 1966 called "Psychedelic Agents in Creative Problem-Solving: A Pilot Study."[16] This study was the first of its kind and still stands alone in proving the relationship between psychedelic use at a moderate level and creativity and problem-solving.

I cannot stress enough the importance of James Fadiman's decades-long ripple of influence through the field of psychedelics. There's a good reason he is known as "The Godfather of Microdosing." He formally introduced the term "microdosing" to the psychedelic lexicon and popularized the practice through his book *The Psychedelic Explorer's Guide* in 2011.[17]

Packed with anecdotal reports, breakthrough transformations, and practical tips on how to use microdosing, his book inspired countless others to experiment for themselves. Hundreds of people requested Fadiman's protocol, and many returned reports on LSD and psilocybin, as well as ayahuasca, iboga, and other, more obscure substances like Syrian rue.

## Microdosing Goes Mainstream

By March 2015, Fadiman's work reached a broader audience when he appeared on the massively popular *Tim Ferriss Show* podcast. With its wide and relatively mainstream appeal—covering business, "biohacking," personal development, exercise, and spirituality, among other topics—the podcast appearance marked a turning point in the microdosing movement. No longer the exclusive domain of the psychedelic fringe, now some of the most influential people in the world, including venture capitalists and tech entrepreneurs, were in on it. As others reported on the trend, microdosing only continued to grow in popularity.

The initial wave of media coverage focused primarily on the benefits of microdosing. This was due to the trend of successful engineers, entrepreneurs, and high-powered Silicon Valley types touting the use of psychedelics to improve productivity.

A *GQ* story claimed, "micro-dosing had made [the subject's] thinking clearer, allowing him to make better connections between his thoughts and words. The difference was manifest in the way he wrote. With a microdose of LSD, he felt abnormally productive, quick, and clever in emails."[18]

In Portland, an article in *Willamette Week* suggested that thousands of people from many walks of life were microdosing with LSD or psilocybin.[19] "We've had dentists and doctors, professional musicians, students, of course, and everyday regular lower-wage [workers]," a woman named Helen said of a new psychedelic research and exploration group. "Really, I don't see any kind of trend in terms of profession."

Pro-microdose evidence has been accumulating. For example, in 2016, *Psychedelic Press, Volume XV* finally published Fadiman's Phase I research, along with a list of conditions people had successfully treated with microdosing.

The January 2017 publication of Ayelet Waldman's *A Really Good Day: How Microdosing Made a Mega Difference in My Mood, My Marriage, and My Life* further catalyzed the spread of microdosing's appeal, this time from the relatively niche biohacking crowd to the realm of the stay-at-home mom. Crucially, Waldman reframed microdosing as a tool for mental health—not merely a billionaire's plaything. Within the broader context of mainstream medical marijuana and the FDA's designation of MDMA and ketamine as "breakthrough therapies," it was an idea whose time had come.

Subsequent media coverage focused more on the therapeutic applications of microdosing and psychedelics in general.

A piece in *The New Yorker* profiled Waldman as a productive, middle-class wife and mother who, having tried many other treatments without success, finally turned to LSD as a way of saving her relationship with her family.[20] The article also emphasized the safety of LSD, almost without reservation, and practically lamented its illegality. Other reports—in *Mashable*, *The Economist*, *HuffPost*, *Crave*, *Willamette Week*, and the *BBC*, among many others—took a similarly sympathetic approach to microdosing and the people who do it.[21]

The fact that microdosing has become almost normalized in the media has thankfully led to more nuanced coverage. There have been several excellent pieces that feature Third Wave and my work specifically. In 2017, *Quartz* published an article titled "How Microdosing Psychedelics Like LSD Could Boost Your Leadership Skills."[22] In this interview, I discussed how people in traditional work environments, tired of the adverse side effects of coffee and Adderall, often find microdosing psychedelics helpful for prosocial tendencies.

*Rolling Stone's* September 2017 piece looked closely at the one-to-one coaching services I offered via Skype while barely mentioning the controversy and novelty of microdosing itself—the media's earlier preoccupation.[23]

In early 2020, the *BBC* did a piece on the longer-term impacts of microdosing.[24] The reporter came along for an in-person session I had with a client. While my client was microdosing, we walked through the redwood forests near Oakland and discussed his purpose, mission, and life path. The article gives an insider view of this work and highlights the burgeoning intersection between psychedelics and coaching. People are becoming more open to coaching and therapy in general, and they're interested in how psychedelics can be a catalyst in these environments to accelerate behavioral change.

Today, many microdosing enthusiasts have congregated on Reddit, participating in a subreddit with more than 200,000 subscribers as of June 2022.[25] People on the forum discuss all aspects of microdosing, including dosage, substances, and results. A poster who took microdoses of psilocybin for seven weeks, for example, reported results like the accounts showing up in news stories. "My focus on work ability increased dramatically (and has been almost since the beginning)," the poster wrote. "My work mood has improved too. I keep brief notes about how I feel, from grumpy to meh to good, and almost every day is good."[26] The majority of these anecdotal reports—at least on the internet —fall somewhere between cautiously optimistic and eagerly instructive.

In one post, users talked about how microdosing did (or did not) help them solve math problems. "I do very abstract maths daily (I'm in academia), and for me, microdosing seems to help with the creative problem-solving aspect but makes me slightly worse at tedious calculations/brute-force proofs," a poster wrote.

"I'm in engineering," another added, "and it really helps me tackle a problem in creative ways if I find old methods don't work."[27]

## A Resurgence of Research

Perhaps unsurprisingly, we're now seeing serious microdosing research by major institutions, with millions of dollars of funding and dozens of studies published. The Beckley Foundation and Imperial College London, for example, crowdfunded a brain-imaging study to measure pattern recognition and creativity on microdoses of LSD.[28] The Australian Research Council's Centre of Excellence in Cognition and its Disorders (ARC CCD) carried out an online survey of microdosers paid for by the Australian government.[29] Other institutions, including MAPS, NYU, and Johns Hopkins, have continued to research the broader utility of psychedelics at higher doses. According to Fadiman, double-blind microdosing studies using placebos could eventually pave the way for FDA approval.[30]

Research on microdosing is quickly gaining traction, and researchers are consistently publishing new studies on overall efficacy, pros and cons, and the potential placebo effect, among other things. Research and experimentation on microdosing are in their infancy, and despite its popularity, it only constitutes a minority of psychedelic research.

When Third Wave began, there was a lack of qualitative research in the scientific community. We relied on reports of user experiences from Reddit and case studies we'd done at Third Wave to show the effects and efficacy of microdosing.

For example, I have personally had very positive results from infrequent psilocybin microdosing. I have found fast and relatively long-lasting relief from depression and social anxiety from doing this, as compared to other pharmaceutical options I've been offered such as SSRIs (selective serotonin reuptake inhibitors). I particularly appreciate the impact and assistance psilocybin offers without the (for me) intolerable side effects.

Further, I feel more open to other people. When I'm at home with my family, I not only feel better equipped to deal with disagreements, I also more often take the initiative to talk. I've found my emotional reactions are less automatic, my mood improves, and I have better contact with my feelings and less restlessness.

Of course, experiences like mine are shared anecdotally. That's why, in part, it is so exciting to know that today, substantial observational research backs up our mission. A great example of this is "Powerful Substances in Tiny Amounts: An Interview Study of Psychedelic Microdosing" by Petter Johnstad, published in 2018.[31]

Similarly, the 2019 publication "Psychedelic Microdosing Benefits and Challenges: An Empirical Codebook" provides an overview of the various aspects that microdosing may affect, such as mood, cognition, and anxiety.[32] In developing the Empirical Codebook, the researchers created a blueprint that other researchers can use in further experimentation. The observational research chronicled in this publication will improve the overall methodology in the future of microdosing research. That's a win for everyone.

Another broad-brushstroke qualitative study to inform future experimental research is "A Systematic Study of Microdosing Psychedelics," published in 2019.[33] This study dives deeper into the pros and cons of microdosing, and its research will help serve as the foundation and clarify hypotheses for future studies.

Finally, perhaps nothing could be more indicative that we are indeed experiencing the psychedelic Third Wave than the business world's piquing interest in these important substances. Companies are being started and structured around experimental microdosing research. Two current examples are MindMed, which is researching microdosing for treatment of ADHD, and Diamond Therapeutics, which is researching psilocybin microdosing for mood enhancement and the treatment of depression.

## Democratizing Psychedelic Medicine

Since the first edition of this book was published, the media's portrayal of psychedelics has shifted significantly. This is mostly due to the overwhelming research helping to define them as helpful medicine. In fact, almost all media is now coming out in support of psychedelics. The focus is much less around the "bad drug" narrative or the "debauchery" narrative leftover from The Summer of Love.

For example, author Michael Pollan, famous for his books on the history, culture, and ethics of food production, contributed a considerable advancement to the mainstreaming of psychedelics with a 2015 *New Yorker* article about research on psilocybin for end-of-life anxiety. Entitled "The Trip Treatment", it was an appetizer to his later *New York Times* number one best-selling book

*How to Change Your Mind*, which transformed the culture's understanding of the potent possibilities associated with psychedelics.[34]

The general perception of psychedelics has done such a 180-degree turn that a current criticism stems not from its former status as a "bad drug" but rather from concerns over its equal distribution. One prevailing note of criticism is that LSD is a gentrified drug.[35] The situation in Silicon Valley, where we see well-paid, mostly White tech guys using a drug to boost their productivity and "become better capitalists," reinforces this view. The concern is that, in no time, those from lower socioeconomic statuses who need this important medicine won't be able to afford it.

I call bullshit. This perspective is fundamentally at odds with how the psychedelic space is developing, as such a viewpoint completely overlooks efforts to decriminalize all plant medicines. These decriminalization laws contain clear stipulations to prevent the commercial sale of the medicines themselves. Eventually, one might be able to legally charge for a ceremony or a guided experience. Still, the legal framework is set up to ensure that these medicines remain accessible to those who need them the most, in both macro and microdoses. These legal developments ensure that these medicines won't become pharma's next big cash cow.

The future of psychedelics isn't just a plaything for any one company or demographic to monopolize. There's a real need for this medicine to reach the greater population. This need drives me to democratize education through the Third Wave. I believe that anyone interested in using psychedelics intentionally and responsibly should be able to easily access information to help them navigate this landscape for free. That is why Third Wave offers top-notch free educational material anyone can access and benefit from.

As consciousness researcher David Jay Brown urged in *The New Science of Psychedelics*: "If we learn how to improve our lives with psychedelics…it's our responsibility, our sacred duty, to share what we've learned with the rest of the world."[36]

And there truly are a myriad of benefits to share.

## The Benefits of Microdosing

The sheer number and depth of benefits ascribed to microdosing are astounding. They seem to cover the whole gamut of human experience, from the minutiae of everyday life to great philosophical insights. Here, I must caution you that you are not guaranteed to experience all, or indeed any, of these benefits. But many people do, so it's worthwhile to outline them.

At Third Wave, we have heard directly from participants about why they pursued microdosing and what they hoped to gain from it. Their answers confirmed what we had been seeing and talking about for years: there are as many motivations for microdosing as there are people on earth. In one survey, evenly spread between the ages of eighteen and seventy-five, most participants hoped that microdosing could help them with at least one of the following:

- Professional development
- Finding purpose
- Increasing energy, focus, and motivation, or overcoming procrastination
- Enhancing or reawakening creativity
- Opening up to others and improving relationships
- Nurturing self-acceptance
- Finding general contentedness
- Letting go of bad habits
- Overcoming fears
- Attaining self-realization
- Improving mental health
- Optimizing athletic performance

Additionally, many were simply curious to see what microdosing could do for them or what it would feel like, as they were intrigued by the positive media coverage.

My initial expectations for microdosing ran in parallel. Specifically, I wanted to reach a flow state that would allow me to become more productive. I wanted to stop procrastinating and grow my online teaching business. I also wanted to reduce my social anxiety so I could more easily connect with others. For those reasons alone, microdosing seemed like a "life hack" worth trying.

## Deeper Sense of Connection

Like so many others, what I gained was far more useful and transformative than expected. Yes, I saw an end to my social anxiety and insecurities, but I also developed more empathy and compassion, experienced deeper engagement in my relationships, and was able to cultivate a sense of presence that I'd rarely felt before.

Even better, microdosing also shed light on points of vulnerability that I didn't even know were there.

Microdosing helped me become aware of the source of my social anxiety. I've always been an introvert who needs time to recharge between social engagements. Like many, I'd tried to tame that social anxiety with alcohol, which was more detrimental than helpful. Microdosing helped me foster prosocial qualities by stripping away the pretense from my interactions that would typically leave me drained; it brought ease and depth to my communications.

Microdosing also helped me understand who I am as a person. I was able to accept my naturally introverted side and reframe it as something to leverage rather than repress. I stopped being so hard on myself when I realized I needed to recharge. I developed the confidence and patience to prioritize rest so I could show up with more presence when with others. I was able to step out of the story that I was "socially awkward" and allowed myself to show up as my free and authentic self. Once I'd done this, I realized that so many of us are suffering from the fear of being rejected for who we truly are. But for humans, community means survival, and our disconnection from that is detrimental.

This microdosing-induced self-reflection also unearthed some of the unpleasant driving forces behind my desire for increased productivity. When engaging with psychedelics, there tends to be a "deconditioning of the shoulds" and a deeper desire to ask ourselves what we truly want. I examined why I was so driven to perform in the first place. I reevaluated my relationship with work and how my focus on performance was rooted in covering up some deep-seated anxiety about inadequacy. This enabled me to tune in internally and come to some realizations about my true desires, not the "shoulds" that peers, parents, and the broader culture externally impose.

This reevaluation didn't stop me from working. It simply helped me pinpoint a direction that felt authentic for my life. My professional path and my personal mission became inextricably linked with microdosing. The practice helped me understand which projects felt truly aligned with my truth.

When I was building TOEFL Speaking Teacher, I knew I loved education, teaching, and building curriculums, but I also knew I wouldn't teach English for the rest of my life. Instead, I saw it as a stepping stone to something greater: Third Wave. Thanks to a much-improved ability to handle complex tasks and integrate new information, after I grew my online English teaching business, I was able to officially bring Third Wave to the world.

Not long after that, I co-founded a third business, called

Synthesis, a legal, medically supervised psilocybin retreat located in the Netherlands where psilocybin truffles have been legal for years.

Our goal with Synthesis was to weave together ancient modalities with contemporary practices such as coaching, psychotherapy, and music therapy. Synthesis eventually became the gold standard for legal psilocybin retreats globally.

Through Synthesis, I understood how working in person with clients motivated me. During the eight retreats I led at Synthesis in 2018, I learned that I wanted to make human connection a central part of my professional work. I have loved many other aspects of my work: creating courses, doing podcast interviews, thinking about scalable products, and more, but nothing resonates with me on a soul level like human connection.

Since those experiences in 2018, I have continued to move in the direction of human-to-human connection. I credit microdosing not only for helping me understand my core values but also for helping me to stay true to them in my business ventures.

## Mood Boost

Like me, many of Third Wave's podcast guests found that the benefits exceeded their expectations. For example, entrepreneur Janet Chang said she found her productivity to be measurably improved in specific areas, like sales and outreach.[37] However, she experienced vast improvements in several other areas as well, including emotional self-awareness, mood, creativity, and sociability.

Janet's story is a compelling one, and not just because she did such an exemplary job of self-tracking throughout her yearlong experiment with microdosing psilocybin.

Careful to guard against the placebo effect by avoiding others' accounts of their experiences, she tried to be as objective as possible, experimenting with various dosage levels and keeping detailed reports on several key data points. These included the quantity and nature of her thoughts, creativity, and sociability. She also used rankings between 1 and 5 to rate her anxiety, mood, and productivity levels and categorized the numbers as follows:

1. Extremely low
2. Slightly lower than normal
3. Normal (baseline)
4. Slightly higher than normal
5. Extremely high

At 0.15 to 0.2 grams of psilocybin mushrooms (Fadiman's suggested microdose) she experienced mild improvements to her mood and anxiety levels (rated 3.25 and 2.13, respectively) but not to her productivity (which idled at 2.75).

The following dosage level was 0.2 to 0.4 g, and she had the opportunity to test between two different work environments: one less orderly and more social, and the other more organized and mostly independent. In the former environment, she found she was extremely productive (4.71) but also highly anxious (3.43).

In the latter, she was somewhat less anxious (3.17) but also less focused (2.61). Her mood was generally exaggerated, characterized by higher highs and lower lows.

Finally, at 0.5 g, typically described as a "minidose" or "creative dose," Janet was surprised to find her anxiety levels almost negligible at 1.41. (As a sidenote, a "minidose" is a slightly perceptible amount of psychedelic that still allows for normal day-to-day functioning.) Her mood and productivity levels significantly improved at 4.50 and 4.07, respectively.[38]

## Sub-Perceptual Sparkle

For many, microdosing transforms work into a kind of "creative play," as Dr. Fadiman's respondent "Madeline" put it, or "professional satori"—a state in which "you are doing what you do professionally, you are doing it well, time passes quickly, and you are pleased with your output."[39]

Satori is the sense of time dilation we experience while microdosing. This is sometimes called "work flow" or "flow state." While experiencing satori, two hours spent on a task may feel like twenty minutes. A 2019 study provides evidence that LSD influences our perception of time, which increases our sense of flow.[40]

On the other hand, it's important to note that microdosing isn't and shouldn't be seen as a way to make staying on the wrong path less arduous. For example, it doesn't seem reliably useful for getting through work you'd rather not be doing. It simply adds what Third Wave contributor Rosalind Stone describes as a "sub-perceptual sparkle."[41]

In *The Psychedelic Explorer's Guide*, "Charles" recounts becoming aware of the oneness inherent in the world:

> What I feel that microdosing does is to slightly rearrange my neural furniture so that glimmers of full-on psychedelic states are constantly pouring into my awareness. I can see how the spider, her web, the wall the web is on, the house the wall is part of, the town the house is part of, and so on, are all connected. It becomes easy to see those connections, in fact, practically self-evident. And from there, it's just a short step to radically affirming the rightness of the spider's web, just the way it is in this moment.

Respondent "Anita" agreed, finding herself "more able to see the world as interrelated rather than disjointed" on microdoses of psilocybin.

Certainly, this accords with my own experience of microdosing and how it helped to accelerate my progress along the path I was already on, the path that I knew to be right. Far from encouraging me to bypass resistance, microdosing helped identify the various points of internal resistance to growth, and it helped me commit to making the necessary changes.

That's not to say microdosing causes you to live "inside your head." On the contrary, many users find they're more present and better able to respond to the moment's demand. As one of our survey respondents said, "microdosing doesn't allow me to be anywhere but in the present moment....I am incapable of worrying about what's going to happen next week, tomorrow, or even five minutes from now."

As such, microdosers tend to be less critical about themselves and their situation and are generally more content. "What I find is that it's easy for me to appreciate everyone and everything in my life, to easily and naturally step into a space of gratitude and sustain it," said one of Fadiman's sources. A Third Wave community member was more specific, recalling how a pizza he'd ordered many times before somehow tasted like the best he'd had in years after microdosing, giving him a "blissful and grateful feeling."

## Microdosing for Mental Health

The full range of benefits offered by microdosing includes the impact it has on mental health. Already, so many people are turning to microdosing for anxiety, depression, PTSD, OCD, ADD/ADHD, and a range of other conditions, as well as for weaning off conventional medications.

(Note: If you plan to go off your medications, it is best to do so under the supervision of a physician.)

In 2019, a clinical trial was the first to compare three different dosages of LSD: six, thirteen, and twenty micrograms.[42] This study shows that even doses as low as six micrograms have a physiological effect on the body, which means that the benefits of microdosing can't be automatically attributed to the placebo effect. It's the first study of its kind and leaves room for interpretation and further research, but it establishes that there is a dose-response for microdoses.

## Depression and Anxiety

By now, the ability of a full dose of psychedelics such as LSD and psilocybin to help treat and alleviate mental disorders such as depression and anxiety is well-established. Numerous studies have suggested that these substances can help people confront and move past their suffering, even when conventional methods of treatment and pharmaceutical interventions such as SSRIs have failed.

Though we don't know precisely how microdosing helps people reduce or eliminate reliance on pharmaceutical pills, it's a promising area of research. Indeed, we don't know how most conventional psychiatric medicines work, how to predict what dose is appropriate, or when they can be most effectively deployed.[43] The side effects of these ubiquitous medications are known, however, including insomnia, drowsiness, and problems with sexual function.

None of these are side effects of microdosing psychedelics.

Because conventional medical treatments are insufficiently understood, many psychiatrists essentially take a shotgun approach to their practice, putting patients on several pills at once in the hope that one of them, or some combination, can help. Often, it doesn't help. One study found that certain SSRIs such as Paxil and Prozac had the same effect on depression as giving patients a sugar pill; in other words, they failed to outperform a placebo.[44] In antidepressant clinical trials conducted by Massachusetts General Hospital and Harvard Medical School, 30 to 40 percent of the subjects responded positively to a placebo.[45]

In the book *Anatomy of an Epidemic*, author Robert Whitaker suggests that our pharmaceutical-first regime of treating mental disorders fails to help people recover over the long-term, and actually increases the chances that people will become dependent on drugs. As the prescribing of pills has skyrocketed, the number of people diagnosed with disabling psychiatric problems has also gone through the roof—from 355,000 in 1955 to over 4 million as of 2007, Whitaker writes.[46]

Recent research compared pharmaceutical models of support to psychedelic healing models of support and found that because SSRIs aim to numb a person's response to their depression, they are effective in the short term at relieving symptoms of depression. The pharmaceutical companies have us all conditioned to seek a quick fix, and by that standard, SSRIs are an effective tool. If a person is feeling suicidal, then the immediate numbing effect of pharmaceuticals may very well save their life. In the long-term, however, their efficacy is no better than placebo.[47]

By contrast, psychedelic users report that rather than having a numbing effect, psychedelics often jumpstart a catharsis and profound personal reckoning that helps them heal the root of their problem. Psychedelics have potential as a longer-term cure.

For those interested in using psychedelics for general relief from depression and anxiety, it's important to understand that the experience and process may be initially harder, as psychedelics often force us to confront challenging emotions like sadness, grief, and anger. But it is only through catharsis that healing can begin. The opportunity and the challenge with psychedelic use is that it requires courage to go into the darkness and meet whatever needs to be faced.

Many readers were up for this challenge of diving into the shadow side and reported success in their attempts to treat certain mental disorders with microdosing. Out of 51 responses to one survey, 60.8 percent said that microdosing helped with depression, 31.4 percent found relief from general anxiety, and 25.5 percent said that it helped with social anxiety.

On a second survey, 229 respondents gave microdosing an average score of 3.8 on an efficacy scale of one to six for lowering anxiety and 4.1 for reducing depression.

As promising as these numbers are, nothing compares to the words readers use to express their satisfaction:

"Only thing that helped my depression, it's a miracle medicine!" one reader wrote.

"I have a history of anxiety/depression and have found in the past that these symptoms have been more controlled in times that I had experimented with psychedelics," one reader reported. "I had heard about microdosing in the last year or so and thought it would be a logical experiment."

"I have fought depression for some 6–7 years since adolescence, micro-dosing has, so far, consistently helped me get on with my day to day, just as much on no MD days as MD days. This also applies to social & general anxiety which has been less severe but experienced for the same period," another reported.

We shouldn't be surprised. Fadiman found that improved mental health, in general, was a common result experienced by microdosers. "It appears that behavior changes were real, observable, and pervasive. Most changes were improvements that reflected increased self-worth, reduced anxiety, and lessened feelings of inadequacy," he wrote in his book, *The Psychedelic Explorer's Guide.* "In addition, the subjects formed deeper and more meaningful relationships."[48]

Fadiman and his co-researcher Sophia Korb presented some of the preliminary results of a new study on microdosing at Psychedelic Science 2017, a gathering sponsored by the Multidisciplinary Association for Psychedelic Studies (MAPS). "The largest group of people who write to us are people with depression and treatment-resistant depression," Fadiman said to the MAPS audience. Out of an initial 418 respondents, 35 percent cited depression as the reason they began microdosing, and 27 percent cited anxiety. In contrast, 58 percent said they were motivated by a combination of both depression and anxiety.[49]

In another survey Fadiman conducted, respondents reported that after microdosing, they experienced an overall increase in feelings of determination, activity, alertness, strength, and enthusiasm, with a decrease in feelings of depression, disturbance, guilt, and fear.

How did microdosing accomplish all of this? Korb shared the insights of people with treatment-resistant depression who found microdosing helpful. "I have noticed that my 'mental chatter' is considerably less than it was prior to this study," one respondent wrote. "I'm feeling very focused, very energetic, very alert," another said. One participant said, "My self-talk feels like from a third-person view."

Your mileage, of course, may vary, and some people reported that microdosing made their mental health problems worse. For example, some who were trying to treat anxiety reported to Fadiman that microdosing increased, rather than decreased, their anxious feelings. In that same vein, a Third Wave reader reported that microdosing heightened anxiety "when combined with excessive caffeine." Another reader wrote: "Can enhance paranoia, be careful."

Yet many more Third Wave readers have praised microdosing for its effect on both depression and anxiety: "I overcame my depression with microdosing because I can consistently be productive and happy with it as a creative booster," one reader wrote. "It also eliminates any anxiety I get because I never used to raise my hand in class. I smoke a lot of cannabis and it's unhealthy to overindulge. I found microdosing to make me feel the need to be productive so I smoke much less when I microdose and don't indulge just to smoke."

Another respondent had a similar experience: "Happiness and sense of gratitude was pervasive and extended into personal life creating a quiet sense of well-being—anti-depression. General anxiety and stress decreased for the most part."

"I can function without anxiety for the first time in years," a survey participant reported to Third Wave. "I feel that my attention span is greater, I'm concentrating like never before. When I was suffering with pain I was given a lot of prescription pain pills and was quickly becoming addicted to them. Microdosing instantly helped me stop taking the several pills a day I was taking just so I could get out of bed, and I haven't touched them since."

In a powerful statement, a Third Wave reader shared a similar anecdote about a life-saving experiment with microdosing:

Immediately I felt less anxiety. The little things I worried about on a day to day basis, didn't worry me anymore. I was able to recognize how "little" they actually were for the first time ever. I felt more connected to the universe and experienced an overwhelming amount of peace. I was in a lot of pain at the time I tried microdosing. I was taking an obscene amount of pain pills and I knew it was only a matter of time before I would have to try something stronger and it scared me. The first time I microdosed I felt like I wasn't going to die anymore. For several weeks leading up to me microdosing I was convinced that whatever I was experiencing was going to kill me. After the mushrooms kicked in for the very first time I wasn't afraid of dying anymore. I believed that no matter what was going to happen that I was going to be ok. Microdosing saved my life.

A study published in November 2021 looked at microdosing practices, motivations, and mental health among a sample of over nine thousand people.[50] In this sample, psilocybin was the most commonly used substance, often "stacked" with other substances, such as lion's mane, cordyceps, niacin, ashwagandha, rhodiola, and others. The core finding of this study was that most of the participants who microdosed showed lower levels of depression and anxiety and were motivated to take responsibility for their health and well-being.

Taking responsibility for one's well-being is an operative concept here. Microdosing isn't a magic pill, even though it can be used as a catalyst to weave in new behavioral change. Any microdosing protocol must be rooted in intention and outcome. That means being proactive to make sure you are supporting yourself in four core areas: a healthy diet, adequate sleep, exercise, and practices for emotional well-being, such as meditation or therapy. When we experience relief, often we look to the tangible thing that's changed in our routines—in this case, the psilocybin—and we give it sole credit for our improvements. But it wasn't simply the substance that caused these changes. It was an exponential combination of all the habits that microdosing facilitated coming together to support us in all the right ways.

Those four key areas are essential on the individual level, but there is another element that microdosing unlocks for many people: community. We're learning that many people benefit from microdosing by experiencing ease in prosocial behaviors, like my personal story of embracing my introversion and thereby making my interactions more meaningful and connective.

Many reports assert that the key to the power of psychedelics is improved self-awareness. One respondent to a Third Wave survey said as much:

> I became much more self-aware and willing to look at my short-comings and character defects in a non-judgmental way. Example: I noticed that when I couldn't control a situation that I would get very anxious. An hour later as I was observing my mental focus on this, and some physical reactions to this, I began to have a dialogue with myself to understand why this was happening. I realized that it is completely human to want to be in control of everything. I told myself that the beauty in this is that I am not in control of what goes on around me and this was a big relief. I also noticed that it took a little time to start noticing these things fully. This was a JOURNEY with curves and a lot of learning about myself which I am grateful for.

Accounts in popular media have also supported the notion of microdosing helping people with anxiety and depression. In the 2015 *Rolling Stone* piece that kicked off the wave of reporting on microdosing, Fadiman's positive results were cited. "His correspondents have told him regular microdosing has alleviated a bevy of disorders, including depression, migraines and chronic-fatigue syndrome, while increasing outside-the-box thinking," the article states.[51]

An article in Portland's *Willamette Week* describes a middle-aged mother and musician. "She suffered from anxiety and PTSD from childhood trauma that was so severe she could no longer perform," the story says, "but taking low-dose mushrooms gave her the fortitude to get back onstage."[52]

## Physical Health

Some people have managed physical issues through microdosing, including chronic pain, migraines, and menstrual cramps. This relief has been known to outlast the protocol itself.[53]

People commonly report a general feeling of health and wellness, often rooted in a stronger mind-body connection. Many microdosers have remarked on this. One, mentioned in a 2017 *Economist* article, felt "sharper, more aware of what [the] body needs" on 1P-LSD, while Fadiman's respondent "Madeline" felt "so healthy and connected to [her] body" that she began to cry.[54]

Athletes often appreciate the physical effects of microdosing, whether they participate in team sports or other physical activities, such as yoga, martial arts, or dance. One Reddit user—a professional dancer—reported improvements in balance, stamina, energy, and a far greater sense of interconnectivity between the muscles.[55] Others have reported stamina boosts for cycling, running, and other exercises.[56] "Within an hour after I swallow my [microdose], I start feeling more energy," wrote one of Fadiman's sources. "It's a kind of bubbling burning on a very low level; my

cells and systems are pumped up with a noticeable kind of buzz...
What's lovely is that it's a kind of good secondary energy, that is,
I can use it to work out with weights, do Pilates, ride my bike, or
really just enjoy being with my body."

Another source, who microdosed psilocybin for surfing, said,
"I was so much more in my body and could feel deeper into it. I
sensed the wave had come thousands of miles and that we were
coming together for its last few seconds before it hit the beach.
But what was best was feeling like I connected back into the
greater world."[57]

A common reported experience for folks who are microdosing
is that it tends to have a harmonizing effect on the body. Women
in particular report that microdosing can have a positive effect
on painful menstrual cramps.[58] Microdosing also helps with pain
tolerance, which may explain some of the alleviation women experience
while menstruating.[59] Researchers studying microdosing on
chronic pain found that microdoses allowed people to withstand
pain longer.

When we look at the intersection of microdosing and neuroplasticity, we see that pain can lead to more neural pathways that
create more pain. Microdosing LSD can interrupt these patterns
and stop compounding chronic pain. It allows people to take a step
back from the experience, which can reduce the overall intensity. If
someone consistently experiences painful menstruation or chronic
back pain but then microdoses, they can interrupt the pattern and
rewire the brain to shift its overall perception. After all, a lot of

pain is psychosomatic. That doesn't mean that it isn't genuine or that people are not truly experiencing it; it just means that it may not be solely coming from the body. That means it is possible to interrupt the signal.

## The Effect Is in the Dose

When I interviewed him for the Third Wave podcast in early 2021, Dr. James Fadiman drew an interesting historical parallel between psychedelics and aspirin.[60] Aspirin was used in very high doses by indigenous people to relieve pain and fever. Then about a hundred years ago, someone discovered that taking low doses of aspirin consistently can reduce health risks associated with heart disease. Here was a medicine historically used in macrodoses, and by slightly altering its method of consumption, we discovered a novel application that helped people in new ways.

Microdosing psychedelics is similar. Yes, there are overlaps in the benefits between micro and macrodosing, but microdosing opens a new understanding of different applications of the same drug that we wouldn't necessarily apply to higher doses.

Fadiman describes the effects of macrodosing and microdosing through a radio metaphor, where one is the AM dial and the other is the FM dial. Both macrodosing and microdosing assist in tuning into a frequency of higher consciousness, in the same way that both dials allow us to access radio frequencies. But different-sized doses create unique waves of experience.

While both macrodosing and microdosing aim toward the same goals—health, balance, and resolution of core issues—they create very different experiences. And, in my opinion, one has way more potential to flourish in today's society.

Indeed, several Third Wave readers reported that they decided to try microdosing specifically because they wanted a new avenue to help mitigate depression and anxiety-related issues.

Microdosing is the way forward. It helps people heal the root issues of what they're struggling with, but it does so in a way that is much less intense, less overwhelming, and has less potential for a retraumatizing experience.

All microdosing compounds affect neurotransmitters in the brain but to different degrees. Your specific goals can make a big difference when choosing to microdose with LSD or psilocybin.[61]

LSD is more dopaminergic, meaning it has more of an effect on dopamine production, while psilocybin is more serotonergic, meaning it has more impact on serotonin production. What that means in practice is that LSD tends to work better to treat depression and psilocybin tends to work better to treat anxiety. People trying to manage their anxiety through microdosing sometimes report that LSD makes their anxiety worse.

This maps pretty well onto what we know about how these different compounds affect the neurobiology of our brains. Therefore, we can predict the best use case for these substances because we know how they affect neurotransmitters. If someone is feeling very low energy, microdosing LSD—a dopaminergic—is more beneficial to get them out of that low-dopamine rut than psilocybin.

Conversely, serotonergic psilocybin helps people feel more grounded, embodied, and intentional, which is more helpful with managing anxiety.

## Where Microdosing Helps Most

### The Professional Sphere

It's no coincidence that many people working in high-stakes business environments, such as Silicon Valley startups, turn to microdosing, intending to enhance creativity and flow. At the same time, many publications—alongside our surveys from Third Wave readers—find that mental health issues—particularly depression—pervade environments where people are putting in impossibly long hours under the pressure of knowing that most startups fail to become sustainable businesses.

Nearly half the entrepreneurs who responded to one such Third Wave survey reported some type of mental health condition. One reason microdosing is so prevalent in Silicon Valley may be that it allows hard-working professionals to manage struggles with depression in a healthier and more productive manner.

Not only do these pressure-cooker conditions contribute to anxiety and depression, but the stigma against showing any sign of perceived weakness is strong in the startup world. For that reason, most people don't talk about it. They recognize that discussing mental health issues could jeopardize funding from investors who might view mental health issues as a risky variable.[62]

Another reason high-tech startups have high rates of depression and anxiety is that they attract certain personalities. For example, in some cases, the very neural atypicalities that help coders develop innovative solutions and display unflagging endurance can also influence their mental health. "Many of the personality traits found in entrepreneurs—creativity, extroversion, open mindedness and a propensity for risk are also traits associated with ADHD, bipolar spectrum conditions, depression and substance abuse," notes a CNN story about the suicide of Eric Salvatierra, a former executive at eBay, PayPal, and Skype.[63]

Leaders in these businesses can improve the situation for themselves and their employees through microdosing. I'm confident that microdosing facilitated my own leadership development. This result can seem surprising at first glance—less so if we consider that leadership straddles the boundary between professional and personal development. Great leadership draws on openness, receptivity, engagement, trust, empathy, and compassion—all of which may be developed through microdosing.

Mindfulness and self-reflection—that is, awareness of our motivations and emotions—are critical elements of good leadership. Without these elements, you can't make wise decisions. Again, these are qualities enhanced by microdosing. Many people who microdose find themselves face-to-face with surprising emotions that previously lay hidden beneath the surface.

## The Personal Sphere

Of course, microdosing for mental health isn't just for Silicon Valley workers or the professional sphere. As I mentioned in the last chapter, the biggest splash in the public consciousness regarding microdosing as a tool to battle mental disorders was over personal relationships and family life. When Ayelet Waldman published *A Really Good Day: How Microdosing Made a Mega Difference in My Mood, My Marriage, and My Life* in 2017, she wrote about losing control of her moods and alienating her family until she found relief through microdosing LSD.[64]

"I believe that these drugs have great therapeutic potential," Waldman said during a podcast interview with Third Wave. "This month changed my life, and I am sad every day that I can't keep doing it legally."[65]

Instantly, Waldman's work was highlighted across the mediasphere. "Countless prescription pharmaceuticals had failed to stabilize her chronic mood disorders, including depression and Bipolar II disorder, and, more recently, her premenstrual dysphoric disorder, a particularly disabling form of premenstrual syndrome," the *New York Times* wrote about her journey. "Her tempestuous psyche, she said, was tearing apart her marriage and raising thoughts of suicide."[66]

"I would have blown up my marriage," she told the newspaper. "I had blown up my marriage. I would have left [her husband] Michael to punish myself. And that's so crazy. All he ever did was love me, and try, but when you love someone who is mentally ill, you're just pouring water into a bucket with a hole in it. It can be exhausting. I think the microdosing actually sealed the hole. Now it's a smaller hole, but we all have to keep on pouring water."

Here's how "sealing the hole" looked for Waldman, as she told the *Guardian:* "Within the first couple of doses, it was like the computer of my brain had been restarted," she said. "I was still moody. I had some really good days, but there were also crappy days, and days when it was just the normal shit. Somehow, though, the bad days were not hellish days, and so I had the capacity to work on issues I just couldn't before. Sure, I was hoping for joy. What I got instead was enough distance from the pain I was in to work on the things that were causing it."[67]

"The horrible crippling depression that I entered the experiment with—that was gone," Waldman said on *The Today Show.* "It allowed me to kind of reset my brain and emotions."[68]

"The mood improvement that coincided with her microdosing changed her whole view of depression," *The New Yorker* weighed in. "It was almost the first time in my life I had perspective on what my moods are," she said to the magazine. "Now, when I slip back into the bad feelings, I know it could get better overnight. And also: there is better."[69]

With Waldman as its avatar, the notion of microdosing became more widespread and popular than ever, and more people became exposed to its potential.

## Want to Go Deeper?

Check out your Microdosing Mastery portal for exclusive resources, articles, and interviews to discover more about the topics from this chapter.

Just go to thethirdwave.co/bonus to access your exclusive book bonuses.

# 3

# Microdosing in the Brain

E arlier, I mentioned that it's not known exactly how psychedelics work in the brain, any more than it's known precisely how medications such as SSRIs work. The science of psychedelics, however, is developing quickly. This chapter will look at where that science has been and where it is going.

The science is still catching up on exactly how microdosing affects the brain, but by taking a critical look at the research out there, we can form a cohesive hypothesis on what is occurring. When I invited neuroscientist Dr. Zach Mainen onto Third Wave's podcast, we talked about how serotonin is likely the key to understanding psychedelics—and how microdosing could affect such powerful transformations in people's lives.

According to Mainen's studies, serotonin is strongly linked to patience and impulse control, adaptability, and neuroplasticity—all effects that microdosers have observed.

Mainen discovered this link through experiments with mice:

In the first experiment, he paired a specific odor with a reward, such as water, to condition the mice to expect that reward whenever they smelled the odor. Later, his team either removed the reward or replaced it with a punishment: a puff of air to the face. Therefore, the mice were compelled to re-associate the odor with a new outcome—a difficult task for any animal since it requires not only overwriting the original association (relearning/plasticity) but also withholding their normal response (impulse control). Mainen found that blocking serotonin receptors made this task even more difficult for the mice.

In the second of Mainen's experiments on mice, he observed their behavior in a controlled environment, first under normal circumstances and then when stimulating serotonin in brief, repeated pulses lasting no longer than a few seconds each. When he stimulated serotonin, the movement of the mice slowed by around half, and they showed fewer signs of jumpiness or impulsivity, an effect supported by numerous other studies.

For microdosers, this is good news. These studies demonstrate the power serotonin has to curb cognitive, knee-jerk reactions to stimuli, which could mean microdosing can help relieve the impulse to pursue harmful addictions or unwanted behaviors.

## Creating New Connections in the Brain

Serotonin is one of the most essential neurotransmitters we have, and it is involved in many diverse functions, including mood, sleep, memory, and cognition. Many antidepressants work by inhibiting serotonin's reuptake (reabsorption) in the brain, thereby increasing its availability.

Serotonin also plays a role in the effects of LSD, psilocybin, and other classic psychedelics, but through a very different mechanism of action. Like serotonin, psychedelics bind to or stimulate serotonin receptors—primarily the subtype known as 5-HT2A.

This leads to (among other things) increases in:

- Production of BDNF (brain-derived neurotrophic factor), a protein that nurtures existing neurons and promotes the genesis of new ones[70]
- Transmission of glutamate, a neurotransmitter involved in cognition, learning, and memory[71]

Although we're still learning about these effects and their interaction with one another, they have clear implications for the potential benefits of microdosing. Many microdosers experience greater neuroplasticity, more rapid learning, and better overall cognitive functioning when committing to a microdosing protocol.

We could hypothesize based on our knowledge that consistent activation of serotonin receptors (including 5-HT2A) through regular microdosing could effectively alter the functioning of the brain. It could potentially deconstruct negative thought patterns and establish new, more beneficial neural pathways.

In addition to influencing serotonin levels, psychedelics may have an impact on stress and well-being. Chronic stress and depression are known to reduce the number of nerve cell connections in the prefrontal cortex. A new study from the Yale University School of Medicine found that a single dose of psilocybin increased both the density and the size of dendritic spines in the prefrontal cortex of living mice.[72] These changes occurred within twenty-four hours and lasted for at least one month afterward. While this study does not deal with microdosing directly, it points to the impact that psilocybin has on the prefrontal cortex and creating new neural connections. It's likely that, when consumed over time alongside a contemplative practice like meditation, an individual microdosing would have a similar outcome. This might explain the patience, receptivity, presence, mindfulness, and adaptability to new ideas that many have seen or experienced from microdosing.

Psychedelics might also disrupt the default mode network (DMN), the part of the brain that is active when people aren't engaged in any particular project or activity. The DMN essentially takes you out of the present moment and triggers daydreams, memory recall, planning for the future, wondering about other people's intentions, and other states that can be useful in some circumstances but can also trap people in persistent patterns of anxiety or depression.[73]

By bypassing old connections in the brain and creating new ones, psychedelics allow people to step away from harmful patterns and nonproductive thoughts and build up a more fruitful state of being.[74]

Disrupting the DMN also helps people be more grounded in the present moment, achieving a state of valuable mindfulness for battling depression.[75] Mindfulness allows people to observe their thoughts and emotions without becoming attached to them, meaning they are less affected by negativity or preoccupations. The state of mindfulness is most commonly associated with meditation, but taking psychedelics can help achieve a similar result, and many people combine both to find peace in their body and mind.[76]

The growing number of studies that show how and why full doses of LSD and psilocybin work to mitigate depression, anxiety, and other mental disorders can help further our understanding of why they could have a similar effect on microdosers.

A groundbreaking clinical study on LSD as a therapeutic modality was published in 2014, the first in four decades. It encompassed four years of data collected between 2008 and 2012 on how the chemical affected anxiety.[77] Twelve participants near the end of their lives were provided LSD-assisted psychotherapy and subsequently interviewed about their responses. The result, the study concluded, was that anxiety "went down and stayed down."

"My LSD experience brought back some lost emotions and ability to trust, lots of psychological insights, and a timeless moment when the universe didn't seem like a trap, but like a revelation of utter beauty," one of the participants said.

Beyond anxiety and depression, other research has shown that psychedelics can also effectively treat substance abuse, perhaps for similar reasons. A 2012 review and meta-analysis of several studies, some conducted in the 1970s or earlier, found that "a single dose of LSD, in the context of various alcoholism treatment programs, is associated with a decrease in alcohol misuse."[78] Anecdotal reports by people who have used psychedelics to combat addiction suggest that feelings of connectivity, gratitude, and beauty have helped them move past their addiction. In other words, people who can address the root causes of problems such as anxiety and depression should have an easier time avoiding getting trapped in cycles of addiction.

Scientists at Imperial College London (ICL) recently produced a study in which they scanned the brains of subjects who had taken LSD, finding a massive boost in connectivity.[79] Researcher Robin Carhart-Harris explained the results:

> Normally our brain consists of independent networks that perform separate specialized functions, such as vision, movement and hearing —as well as more complex things like attention. However, under LSD the separateness of these networks breaks down and instead you see a more integrated or unified brain.

"Our results suggest that this effect underlies the profound altered state of consciousness that people often describe during an LSD experience," Carhart-Harris continued. "It is also related to what people sometimes call 'ego-dissolution,' which means the normal sense of self is broken down and replaced by a sense of reconnection with themselves, others and the natural world. This experience is sometimes framed in a religious or spiritual way—and seems to be associated with improvements in well-being after the drug's effects have subsided."[80]

## Psilocybin Studies

One study, published in 2006, that helped kick off the current wave of psychedelic research, found that psilocybin was helpful to people trying to overcome obsessive-compulsive disorder.[81] The research initially intended to focus on the safety of psilocybin, leaving it up to future scientists to discover its effectiveness, but the positive effects were impossible to ignore. "Marked decreases in OCD symptoms of variable degrees were observed in all subjects during 1 or more of the testing sessions," the study reported. "Improvement generally lasted past the 24-hour timepoint."

Another trial conducted on mice found that animals trained to fear certain stimuli could overcome the fear conditioning more quickly when given low doses of psilocybin.[82]

More recently, a study published in 2016 found evidence that psilocybin could be effective against treatment-resistant depression.[83] Out of twelve subjects who suffered from severe or very severe depression, all showed a reduction in symptoms for at least a week after being administered psilocybin. A majority still felt positive effects three months later. "The magnitude and duration of the post-treatment reductions in symptom severity motivate further controlled research," the study concludes. "Psilocybin has a novel pharmacological action in comparison with currently available treatments for depression and thus could constitute a useful addition to available therapies for the treatment of depression."

A few studies have focused on using psilocybin to reduce anxiety and other problems such as depression and psychological distress in cancer patients. Research carried out at the Harbor-UCLA Medical Center, Johns Hopkins, and New York University found that the substance could have profound and even transformative effects on people facing the end of their lives.

A pilot study at UCLA established that it was safe to administer psilocybin to cancer patients and provided a roadmap forward with results that suggested mood improvement.[84] At Hopkins, 80 percent of participants felt reductions in anxiety and depression after undergoing psilocybin-assisted therapy, and 67 percent went so far as to call it one of the top five meaningful experiences in their lives.[85] "The most interesting and remarkable finding is that a single dose of psilocybin, which lasts four to six hours, produces enduring decreases in depression and anxiety symptoms, and this may represent a fascinating new model for treating some psychiatric conditions," said researcher Roland Griffiths.

NYU reported similar results, concluding the treatment "produced rapid and sustained anxiolytic and antidepressant effects (for at least 7 weeks but potentially as long as 8 months), decreased cancer-related existential distress, increased spiritual well-being and quality of life, and was associated with improved attitudes towards death... Psilocybin, administered in conjunction with appropriate psychotherapy, could become a novel pharmacological-psychosocial treatment modality for cancer-related psychological and existential distress."[86]

One of the study subjects at UCLA, neuropsychologist Annie Levy, spoke of her battle with ovarian cancer and how psilocybin helped her come to terms with her fear. "As soon as it started working I knew I had nothing to be afraid of because it connected me with the universe," she said of her experience, saying she was then able to better see and appreciate her relationships with her loved ones.

"I would recommend psilocybin treatment for anyone with a terminal or potentially terminal illness," she said. "It's more helpful than any other treatment I've ever had."[87]

Lauri Kershman, MD, was a leukemia patient who took psilocybin as part of the Johns Hopkins study. "The impact that the study had on my life was enormous," she said. "The safety that I felt to be able to let go and face some demons and go deep into some pretty difficult and sad places."[88]

Just as it has for LSD, The Imperial College of London has used brain scans to help understand how psilocybin affects the brain. One study revealed how psilocybin facilitates neural connections that are otherwise not present or neglected.[89] "A simple reading of this result would be that the effect of psilocybin is to relax the constraints on brain function, ascribing cognition to a more flexible quality, but when looking at the edge level, the picture becomes more complex," the study's discussion section states. "The brain does not simply become a random system after psilocybin injection, but instead retains some organizational features, albeit different from the normal state, as suggested by the first part of the analysis. Further work is required to identify the exact functional significance of these edges."

Another brain mapping study at ICL found that psilocybin helped stimulate activity in the hippocampus and anterior cingulate cortex, parts of the brain linked to emotional thinking that are often active during dreams.[90] "What we have done in this research is begin to identify the biological basis of the reported mind expansion associated with psychedelic drugs," researcher Carhart-Harris said of the study. "I was fascinated to see similarities between the pattern of brain activity in a psychedelic state and the pattern of brain activity during dream sleep, especially as both involve the primitive areas of the brain linked to emotions and memory. People often describe taking psilocybin as producing a dream-like state and our findings have, for the first time, provided a physical representation for the experience in the brain."

## Fear Is the Opposite of Freedom

Mystical experiences from my early psychedelic journeys helped me recognize the illusion of death, liberating me from the fear of the "other side." An extension of this core fear shows up in how we value our status in society. Throughout history, rejection from the group could mean death for a human, so we've come to fear rejection almost as fervently as we fear death. In the same way psychedelics remove the fear of death, they also remove the fear of rejection. By eliminating fear and "killing" the ego we've created to protect our personality, we allow for greater alignment with our true passions, which often results in a more satisfying relationship with our communities.

Let's explore this idea through the lens of indigenous use. Indigenous use almost always involves macrodosing as a tool of initiation. Through a psychedelic experience, the boy, liberated from his immature ego, is ushered into manhood. Through this ego death, there is a process of transformation that allows the man to come into his true being and be fully seen by his community. Going forward, the man is not concerned about his own egoic needs. Instead, he realizes his contribution is more significant than the wants of the "I".

The effect is not so different in modern culture. We're mainly driven by external sources and seek validation through a strict schedule of life milestones. When we experience ego death, we come to two conclusions: (1) the old part of me has died and now I am reborn, and (2) now that I have been through this kind of death, I know it is nothing to be feared. There is a capacity to see outside the narrow lens of the ego's superficial desires and step into a desire to create, recognizing that the creation contributes to the greater whole.

Fear is the opposite of freedom. The more we live in fear, the less space we experience in everyday life. The less fear we have, the more we can be courageous in the ways we engage with our lives. We can be present in the moment as it emerges and fearlessly create what we want to make.

In psychedelics, we have a medicine that helps us to experience less fear, extending freedom to all aspects of our lives: our interiority, our connection with others, our romantic relationships, our professional aspirations, our harmony with nature, and on and on, so that our lives aren't dictated by our conditioning, but, instead, by the truths we feel compelled to create from.

## Want to Go Deeper?

Check out your Microdosing Mastery portal for exclusive resources, articles, and interviews to discover more about the topics from this chapter.

Just go to thethirdwave.co/bonus to access your exclusive book bonuses.

# PART II

# How to Microdose

# 4

# Cautions, Contraindications, and the Changing Legal Landscape of Microdosing

Transformational experiences like those described in the previous chapters have attracted interest in microdosing. But this widespread media attention has also resulted in a glut of reactionary headlines—often unsubstantiated by the articles themselves—linking microdosing to the risk of death and even acid "flashbacks," among other things.

These claims are primarily baseless, but that doesn't mean we should ignore the potential dangers. Microdosing is a (relatively) new and understudied trend, and there's a need for more research into the side effects and risks of microdosing. But there are some things we already know. This chapter will look at reasons for caution in microdosing and offer tips for avoiding possible pitfalls.

Keep in mind, however, that I'm not a scientist or a physician, and the long-term effects of microdosing have never been studied in detail. As more people experiment with microdosing, our body of knowledge grows. As Dr. Fadiman puts it, we're gradually filling in a map of an otherwise vast, uncharted territory, relying heavily on anecdotal reports from those who have gone before us.

## Legality

Currently, the most obvious drawback to microdosing with psychedelics—and arguably the most significant risk—is that you will be operating outside the law. Psychedelics, especially LSD, tend to be illegal regardless of growing evidence to support these substances' relative safety and therapeutic utility. In a brief editorial piece entitled "Tripping up: The real danger of microdosing with LSD," *New Scientist* echoed the views of the broader scientific community by calling out the discrepancy.[91] The piece called for a more pragmatic, evidence-based approach to drug policy, one that accepts that people use drugs whether they're legal. "The risks deserve further attention," the article concludes, "but a serious criminal record shouldn't be one of them."

Legal developments over the past decade signal possible change in how western governments handle LSD cases. For example, in September 2017, Norway's Supreme Court overturned an initial five-month prison sentence for LSD possession, commuting the sentence to forty-five hours of community service.[92] By citing LSD's potential health benefits, this case may set an example for other Western courts to consider.

The legal landscape is rapidly changing. Today, three core movements are developing in the psychedelic ecosystem: medicalization, legalization, and decriminalization. Nevertheless, most Western governments still criminalize psychedelics. Thus, we must see things as they are—for now at least. And as far as the risks of microdosing go, this is one of the few we know for sure.

At present, ketamine has been medically approved by the FDA. Johnson & Johnson's patented version, Spravato, is being prescribed to treat depression. I consider ketamine to be the new medical marijuana because it can be prescribed off-label for such a wide variety of physical conditions. It's the most widely used psychedelic at this time.

MDMA and psilocybin are still awaiting approval. MDMA is currently in phase 3 clinical trials through the nonprofit MAPS. Approval to treat PTSD is expected in 2023, and soon after it will be approved for a range of conditions off-label, making it widely available through clinicians and prescriber networks.

Compass Pathways is studying psilocybin's efficacy at relieving treatment-resistant depression and is currently in phase 2B trials. Psilocybin is also in clinical trials at the Usona Institute for treatment of major depressive disorder. These companies expect psilocybin to be approved by 2025 for clinical use.

This is critical because once these psychedelics are approved, they can be covered under medical insurance, which is a huge step toward more widespread accessibility.

As far as legalization goes, Oregon legalized psilocybin therapy in 2020 under Proposition 109. This allows a provider network in Oregon to prescribe psilocybin for both medical and nonmedical purposes. If you are prescribing psilocybin to an individual, you must be present with them when they take it. So, a practitioner can both prescribe the psychedelic and charge a certain fee to hold space for an experience. The critical distinction between what Oregon is doing and general FDA approval is that the state of Oregon will allow nonmedical providers and clinicians to prescribe psilocybin. In contrast, FDA approval will only enable clinicians to prescribe psilocybin or MDMA.

Several other states are introducing similar bills. This shows the acceptance for clinical use of psychedelic therapy is generating significant momentum. By the end of this decade, most people who live in the United States will have access to some form of legal psychedelic therapy.

The final thing to note about the changing legal landscape is decriminalization. Decriminalization means that the substance becomes the lowest priority for law enforcement. The first city to decriminalize psilocybin was Denver in May 2019. Soon after, the cities of Oakland, Seattle, and Detroit followed suit by decriminalizing all plant medicines including San Pedro, ayahuasca, and iboga.

The model developing around decriminalization is called "Grow, Gather, Gift." People can grow their own medicine, whether psilocybin, San Pedro, or ayahuasca. They can then give it away, but they cannot charge for it. They can, however, charge to hold a ceremony or experience. In some places, the regulations haven't fully formed around this. The upside to decriminalization is widespread accessibility; the downside is that with the unformed and changing rules and regulations, it's hard to determine how certain violations will be handled.

In places with decriminalized plant medicines, several microdosing supplements have popped up and are sold "above ground." The increasing awareness around microdosing and acceptance of psychedelics as medicine has enabled a gray market. These microdosing supplements will only become more widespread and accessible as the decriminalization movement generates momentum.

Even with all these legal improvements, it's still a good idea to be cautious about your communications and who you trust with this information. But don't worry about the government tapping your phone or scanning text messages for mentions of mushrooms: they are much more focused on other illicit drugs tied to criminality, gangs, and potential overdoses (like fentanyl and cocaine).

Aside from the legal aspects, there may be other risks inherent in microdosing, though the general safety of psilocybin and LSD is well established. Well into old age, Albert Hofmann's regular use of LSD didn't seem to do any damage; he died at 102. Furthermore, James Fadiman and Sophia Korb have seen not one case of lasting harm among the respondents to their ongoing microdosing survey. These facts are reassuring, but they are not enough to verify the long-term safety of microdosing. Let's look closer at what we know so far.

## Heart Problems

One recurrent concern, for instance, is that repeated activation of 5-HT2B receptors in the heart could lead to valvular heart disease (HVD), a condition requiring surgery.[93] This was the case among a small number of patients who were prescribed the now-withdrawn drugs fenfluramine/phentermine (fen-phen) and pergolide (Permax) during the 1990s and most of the 2000s. Fen-phen roughly doubled patients' risk of developing HVD after a ninety-day course of treatment at 30 mg/day. Of course, 30 mg is three thousand times as much as the typical microdose of LSD (10 µg)—the probable cause of trouble, if there is one, may be how LSD binds to 5-HT2B receptors keeps it "trapped" inside for many hours, possibly accumulating over time.

Most reports and studies on psychedelics and heart health are limited and inconclusive. Some have reported abnormal heart effects in the shorter term as well. One user who took a moderate microdose of 10 to 15 µg found his heart rate increased immediately, leading to palpitations, pain, and high blood pressure that persisted for months. However, he also had existing anxiety issues; it's unknown whether these symptoms were due to LSD.

Another study looked at the effects of daily microdoses of psilocin (the main psychoactive form of psilocybin) on rats over three months. Although the researchers reported finding "cardiac abnormalities," their methodology was flawed, and the results lacked any statistical context. So, it is doubtful that microdosing causes any cardiac issues, as properly executed scientific studies have found no link. It is also almost entirely unheard of anecdotally, even with people who consume higher doses more regularly.

It is, however, possible that microdosing could exacerbate existing heart conditions. It may not, but as science currently has no conclusive answer one way or another, it is best that people with existing heart conditions be especially cautious—and perhaps even avoid microdosing altogether—until we know more. If this includes you and you plan to try microdosing anyway, it would be wise to avoid combining microdoses with caffeine.

Ultimately, we just don't know much about the long-term cardiac effects of microdosing. The longitudinal effects of microdosing are still largely unknown, so it is good to be aware of that before diving into a microdosing protocol. For this reason, it's best to limit your microdosing cycles to no more than ninety days at a time, with at least two rest days between each dose and perhaps a month or so between each cycle.

In my personal and observational experience, this consistent three-month cycle helps people get the most out of their microdosing regimen. Just like any other drug that you use regularly, such as caffeine, having a bit of a break from it resets your baseline and makes its effects more potent.

## Contraindications and Possible Interactions

Although microdosing shows excellent potential for treating bipolar depression, individual symptoms and responses will vary. Ayelet Waldman and others may have been able to stabilize their mood swings with LSD. The potential for overstimulation suggests it may be less suitable during the mania phase.

Potential interactions with lithium carbonate, a drug commonly prescribed for bipolar disorder, are incredibly worrying. In his talk at Psychedelic Science 2017, Fadiman made specific reference to this medication, stating that he and Korb were unsure about its safety with microdoses of LSD or psilocybin.[94] Combining lithium with LSD (at macrodoses, at least) can cause seizures and even coma in users with no history of these symptoms—perhaps because both LSD and lithium lower the seizure threshold.

For the same reason, it's probably best to avoid microdosing if you already suffer from seizures. You should also be cautious about combining microdoses with other drugs that appear to lower the seizure threshold. These include certain antiasthmatics, antibiotics, anesthetics, antidepressants, immunosuppressants, and stimulants.[95]

SSRI antidepressants should also be avoided because they lower the seizure threshold and reduce the effects of psychedelics. Common SSRIs include fluoxetine (Prozac), paroxetine (Paxil), sertraline (Zoloft), citalopram (Celexa), and trazodone (Desyrel).

Conversely, monoamine oxidase inhibitors (MAOIs) can significantly *increase* the effects of psychedelics by inhibiting their dissolution in the body. This is why MAOIs are included in the ayahuasca brew. Common MAOIs include the drugs phenelzine (Nardil), isocarboxazid (Marplan), selegiline or L-deprenyl (Eldepryl), moclobemide (Aurorix or Manerix), and furazolidone (Furoxone).

Avoid both MAOIs and SSRIs when microdosing to allow you to maintain control over your microdoses. It's also important to note that SSRIs should not be taken in conjunction with ayahuasca since combining SSRIs and MAOIs can lead to potentially fatal serotonin syndrome.

Iboga is another particularly dangerous psychedelic to combine with other drugs. If you are interested in using it for microdosing, you should check the list of contraindicated medications for any medication you take and always consult with a doctor.[96]

Iboga is a more intense medicine than the other psychedelics. People have suffered cardiac arrests while on large doses of iboga, which doesn't happen with LSD or psilocybin. The protocol for dosing iboga is also different because tolerance builds up quicker. It's more important to take frequent breaks when using iboga.

You may wonder why people gravitate toward iboga when it is more dangerous than other psychedelics. Iboga is a highly effective tool to break opiate addictions because it binds to the same neurological receptors as opiates such as heroin. Still, it is nonaddictive in and of itself.

Another person who may be attracted to iboga is the seasoned microdoser who wants to explore something other than LSD and psilocybin. Even an advanced microdoser will need to integrate more breaks with iboga to avoid building up a tolerance. If you're interested in microdosing with iboga, I cannot stress enough the importance of doing your homework before you begin.

Generally, you should completely wean off all medications before taking it—especially SSRIs/SNRIs. Although relatively little is known about their interaction with iboga, MAOIs should not be taken for at least seven to ten days beforehand. Once again, if you plan to go off your medications, please consult first with a physician.

If you're planning to microdose alongside prescribed medications, it's essential to do your research first. Check with a medical professional and seek advice from others who may be in a similar situation. Our online microdosing course and community at Third Wave are excellent resources to start with.

One final and rather more curious contraindication should be mentioned here: it appears that people with colorblindness often experience visual distortions, including tracers, after taking LSD microdoses. In Korb and Fadiman's research, five participants dropped out because of these effects. It's not clear why colorblind people, in particular, are affected, but if you're one of them, you may want to think twice about microdosing.

## Physical Discomfort

We think of psychedelics first in terms of their effects on our minds, but they also affect the rest of the body. People frequently report muscle cramps after taking LSD microdoses, especially in the neck area, possibly due to vasoconstriction. Taking a warm shower or stretching is said to help. Cramps could also be related to a magnesium deficiency, so magnesium supplements could also be helpful. If the discomfort persists, you should try lowering your dose.

Gastric issues are also somewhat common with psychedelics, primarily LSD and psilocybin. One user who took LSD microdoses on three consecutive days, for example, woke on the second, third, and fourth days with stomach pains or cramps (although this may be due to a change of diet catalyzed by the microdosing mindset). Aside from lowering doses and, in this case, spacing them further apart, ginger tea may help to settle the stomach. With psilocybin mushrooms and other plant material, grinding them up for use in capsules can also avoid gastric upset. I'll cover this in detail in Chapter 7.

## Mood and Energy Effects

As with macrodoses of psychedelics, your mindset going into a microdose could heavily influence the effects. Therefore, you should be cautious about using them during times of stress and upheaval—not least because microdosing can spotlight your thoughts, however positive or negative they may be. While many people find relief from anxiety or depression through microdosing, this amplification of emotional states may be why others find their symptoms aggravated. If you choose to microdose during a difficult time, it may be helpful to meditate, even for just five or ten minutes beforehand.

In our research at Third Wave, we found that if a person doesn't have a grounding practice like meditation, a microdosing protocol can be harmful instead of helpful. Microdosing introduces more chaos into the system; it's a disruptor that helps make things less rigid. These effects can be significant for creativity but bad for existing anxiety.

We recommend that people have a practice to help them integrate this disruption and channel it into a positive outcome. These practices don't need to be advanced. Some of the most effective are classic mindfulness breathing exercises, walking meditations, and focal point exercises. Some people have tried transcendental meditation as well. The more you increase your dose level, the more meditation you should be doing as a balance to the medicine itself. Still, no matter the dosage, mindfulness practice is a key to the efficacy of microdosing.

On the other end of the spectrum, psychedelics can make you feel "too good" in some ways. One user, for example, experienced a stable increase in energy levels and lower anxiety and depression while microdosing psilocybin mushrooms, but when he tried LSD, first at 16 µg and then at 10 µg, he found his energy levels became too high after the first hour. He described his mental state as "scatty" and found it challenging to concentrate on his work and interact with other people. There can be a fine line between high productivity and an inability to focus on any one task. He was also yawning and tired, despite the energy boost. This loss of control, especially at work, could exacerbate anxiety. An obvious solution would be to lower the dose or, if that fails, to stop microdosing altogether.

Some people have trouble sleeping at night, even if they microdose in the morning. This is especially common with LSD due to its longer duration. If you find this a problem, it may be worth switching to psilocybin. On the other hand, microdosing can also lead to fatigue or extreme tiredness when the immediate effects have faded. While some report an afterglow effect that persists for a day or two, others report exhaustion, irritability, and even depression in the days that follow, especially when microdosing more than twice a week. Agitation and irritability appear to be more common with iboga, perhaps because it can accumulate over time in the body.

Some of these effects might point to the need for a change in lifestyle, which is, after all, what microdosing is supposed to assist with. Pay close attention to your diet, sleeping pattern, exercise regimen, and other things affecting your mood and energy levels.

## Impulsivity and Poor Judgment

As author and flow-state authority Steven Kotler said in his Third Wave podcast interview, "the difference between flow and mania is a thin line." In other words, the impulsivity that microdosing gives rise to can be fantastic in many ways—indeed, it's one of microdosing's appeals—but it can also lead to poor judgment and making decisions you may later regret. For example, you might say something you probably shouldn't have, agree to a business project you'd rather have thought more about, or buy unnecessary things that you wouldn't usually buy (something I know all too well from personal experience).

## Inconsistent Effects

Of course, judging how a microdose might affect you is only possible if you know exactly what you're ingesting and how much of it. Unfortunately, you often won't know the precise dose you're taking—especially in the case of LSD, since doses can be considerably more or less potent than advertised. As a result, you may experience inconsistent effects and even full-blown trips, which are problematic if you're at work or driving. That's why it's always essential to start with small doses (5 to 6 μg) and be cautious with each new supply. You should also avoid microdosing at work, especially in potentially hazardous situations, until you're aware of and comfortable with the effects of your dose.

Then again, not knowing the precise dose you're taking is the least of your worries when it comes to sampling new substances. Lack of regulation means you can't even be sure what you're getting. Again, this is especially true in the case of LSD, which is sometimes substituted with the potentially very dangerous 25I-NBO-Me. Many powdered extracts and whole plants, if you're not familiar with them, can easily be mis-sold. There's also the risk of misidentifying substances in the wild—particularly mushrooms, which can be deadly if you get the wrong type. Never harvest wild mushrooms without an expert.

When it comes to herbs and powdered extracts, make sure you're getting a recommendation for a provider from a strong referral that you trust. Legitimate suppliers of herbs and powders that are not psychedelic will state a third party has tested them. A little due diligence goes a long way in ensuring that you're getting the right product.

## Mixing Microdosing
## with Drugs and Supplements

We talked earlier about a few contraindicated medications and substances while microdosing. Happily, the list of medications and supplements that participants in the microdosing study (using

LSD, 1p-LSD, or psilocybin) have reported as having no adverse response is much longer:

Painkillers
- Acetaminophen/paracetamol (Tylenol)
- Aspirin
- Codeine
- Dihydrocodeine (Co-dydramol)
- Hydrocodone (Vicodin, Norco)
- Ibuprofen (Advil, Motrin)
- Naproxen (Aleve)
- Tramadol (Ultram)

Heart/high blood pressure medication
- Amiodarone (Cordarone, Nexterone)
- Hydrochlorothiazide (HCTZ, HCT)
- Lisinopril (Prinivil, Zestril)
- Losartan (Cozaar)
- Spironolactone (Aldactone)
- Telmisartan (Micardis, Actavis)
- Valsartan (Diovan)

Birth control
- Aubra
- Hormonal pills
- Marvelon

- Mirena
- NuvaRing
- Tri-cyclen
- Antacid
- Ranitidine (Zantac)

Antibiotics
- Clindamycin (Cleocin, Dalacin, Clinacin)
- Doxycycline
- Minocycline (Minocin, Minomycin, Akamin)
- Penicillin (Bicillin)
- Antifungals
- Fluconazole (Diflucan, Celozole)

Focus meds (ADHD/ADD)
- Amphetamine (Adderall)
- Bupropion (Wellbutrin)
- Dextroamphetamine (Dexedrine, Metamina, Attentin, Zenzedi, ProCentra, Amfexa)
- Lisdexamfetamine (Vyvanse)
- Methylphenidate (Ritalin, Biphentin)
- Modafinil (Provigil)

Sleep aids
- Zopiclone (Zimovane, Imovane)
- Melatonin

- Zolpidem (Ambien, Stilnox)

Antihistamines
- Cetirizine (Zyrtec)
- Diphenhydramine (Benadryl, Gravol)
- Loratadine (Claritin)
- Ranitidine (Zantac)

Benzodiazepines (Anxiety, sleep, seizure)
- Alprazolam (Xanax)
- Clonazepam (Klonopin)
- Diazepam (Valium)
- Flurazepam (Staurodorm)
- Lorazepam (Ativan)

Other anxiety treatments
- Etizolam
- Propranolol

Parkinson's
- Levodopa
- Pramipexole

Cholesterol
- Atorvastatin (Lipitor)
- Rosuvastatin (Crestor)

- Simvastatin (Zocor)
- Statins
- Racetams
- Aniracetam
- Phenylpiracetam
- Piracetam

Mood stabilizers and antipsychotics
- Aripiprazole (Abilify)
- Buspirone (Buspar)
- lamotrigine (Lamictal)
- Lithium
- Quetiapine (Seroquel)

Diabetes
- Metformin (Glucophage)

Anticonvulsants
- Baclofen (Lioresal)
- Carbamazepine (Tegretol)
- Cyclobenzaprine (Flexeril)
- Gabapentin
- Mirtazapine
- Sodium valproate
- Tizanidine (Zanaflex)

Thyroid
- Methimazole
- Thiamazole

Antidepressants
- Bupropion (Wellbutrin)
- Citalopram (Celexa)
- Desvenlafaxine (Pristiq)
- Doxepin (Sinequan)
- Duloxetine (Cymbalta)
- Escitalopram (Lexapro)
- Paroxetine (Paxil)
- Sertraline (Zoloft)
- Venlafaxine (Effexor)

GERD
- Esomeprazole (Nexium)
- Pantoprazole (Protonix)
- Ranitidine (Zantac)

Breathing (asthma, COPD)
- Salbutamol (Albuterol)
- Cetirizine (Zyrtec)
- Beclomethasone (Clenil Modulite)
- Montelukast (Singulair)
- Antiviral

- Nitazoxanide

Drugs of recreation
- Alcohol
- Amphetamine
- Heroin
- Kratom
- Marijuana
- Nicotine

Anti-inflammatory
- Mesalazine (Octasa)

Immunosuppressant
- Hydroxychloroquine (Quensyl)
- Erectile Dysfunction
- Tadalafil (Cialis)

Alcohol dependence treatment
- Acamprosate (Campral)
- Disulfiram (Antabuse)
- Naltrexone

Hormones and steroids
- Estradiol
- Prednisone (Deltasone, Liquid Pred, Orasone, Adasone, Deltacortisone)

- Estrogen (Premarin)
- Progesterone (Prometrium, Utrogestan, Endometrin)
- Testosterone
- Levothyroxine (Synthroid)
- Nature-Throid
- Dexamethasone
- DHEA
- Spironolactone (Aldactone)

Supplements
- 5-HTP
- Albizia
- Ashwagandha
- B100
- BCAAs
- Biotin
- Brahmi
- Bromelain
- Caffeine
- Calcium
- Cannabis
- Cayenne
- Chaga
- Chlorophyll
- Choline
- CILTEP

- CoQ10
- Cordyceps
- Creatine
- Eleuthero
- EPA/DHA
- Fish oil
- Ginseng
- Glucosamine
- Iodine
- Iron
- Kelp
- Kratom
- L-theanine
- Lemon balm
- Lion's mane
- Maca
- Magnesium
- MCT
- Methyl sulfonyl methane (MSM)
- Milk thistle
- Multivitamins
- Omega 3/6/9
- Passionflower
- Phosphatidyl
- Probiotics
- Pycnogenol

- Reishi
- Rhodiola

Rosacea
- Selenium
- Shatavari
- Skullcap
- St. John's wort
- Taurine
- Tulsi
- Turmeric (curcumin)
- Turkey tail
- Twynsta

Vitamins
- B6
- B12
- C
- D
- D3
- K
- K2
- Zinc
- Zinium

## Weighing the Risks

Microdosing isn't for everybody. Your experience with microdosing psychedelics will always be different from the experiences of others.

To mitigate the downsides as much as possible, keep in mind the following tips:

- Don't microdose at work until you have calibrated your dosage appropriately.
- Start low and go slow, gradually increasing the dose from the minimum.
- Restrict your use to two to three times per week to avoid tolerance buildup and attachment to the effects.
- Limit your protocol to ninety days, and then take a break
- Always test your medicine. We have many LSD testing kit options available at Third Wave.

As we continue to learn how and why microdosing affects people, you can become an early test subject by participating. Only you can decide whether the benefits outweigh the risks—but do so with the understanding that we do not have absolute clarity on the long-term effects.

## Want to Go Deeper?

Check out your Microdosing Mastery portal for exclusive resources, articles, and interviews to discover more about the topics from this chapter.

Just go to thethirdwave.co/bonus to access your exclusive book bonuses.

# 5

# Set Your Intentions

Beginning a microdosing regimen is no casual decision. In committing to transformation with sub-perceptual psychedelics, you're engaging with a tool that offers profound and lasting change. While everybody's experience with microdosing is unique, you can take an active role in shaping your experience by setting clear, tangible intentions before you start.

## Set and Setting

Timothy Leary popularized the phrase "set and setting" in the 1960s as he began to educate a broader populace about psychedelics.[97] "Set" is short for mindset, and "setting" is the physical environment in which the experience occurs, which begs two questions of reflection for you:

1. What is your mindset going into your microdosing experience?
2. And what's the setting you're in? What is the nature of your environment?

These two elements are critical to consider before kicking off any psychedelic experience, much less your microdosing protocol.

Leary based set and setting in his observations of indigenous psychedelic use. As I've previously mentioned, almost all indigenous use is through ritual, often with a shaman present, and always with a certain level of intention and forethought. However, as the Second Wave movement gained momentum, Leary noticed that many folks were using LSD without paying attention to the conditions under which they consumed the medicine and how it impacted their experience. He realized that to protect the integrity of these medicines, he had to educate people on set and setting. In other words, how to clean and stabilize one's mindset going into an experience, and the importance of the specific environment in which the experience takes place.

Psychedelics are nonspecific amplifiers, meaning they don't have inherent values themselves, but they work as a microscope for what's already going on inside your psyche. For instance, if you're going through a particularly challenging time and take LSD or psilocybin, the psychedelic will force you to confront your inner turbulence. If someone expects to trip and experience bliss and love without doing any mindset work beforehand, they may have a rough experience. Similarly, if the setting is chaotic or new or doesn't feel psychologically safe, it's hard to surrender fully, making the medicine less effective.

When preparing for your first microdosing experience, ask yourself:

- What emotions am I experiencing right now? What emotions have I experienced over the past days and weeks?
- What challenges have I come up against in the last several months?
- Is there any trauma that may surface when microdosing with psychedelics?

It's a good idea to talk with a coach, therapist, or guide when exploring these ideas to go into your microdosing protocol with a clear understanding of your internal landscape.

In terms of setting, make sure that the environment you choose is comfortable, familiar, and somewhere you can fully surrender and relax. You also may choose to have a guide present to support you through the experience.

While Leary's parameters for set and setting largely pertain to high doses, I encourage people to abide by these principles even when microdosing, especially when using microdosing as an entry point into an unfamiliar medicine. You never know how sensitive you'll be to a medicine, so don't assume that set and setting won't matter just because you're doing a small dose.

For many, microdosing's lesser intensity holds significant allure because low doses naturally mitigate many of the potential risk factors. Because this is a sub-perceptual dose, you can usually get away with having one element of set and setting that isn't ideal. However, as you scale up the amount of psychedelic you take—and choose to go beyond microdosing—stick by our rule of thumb: the higher the dose, the more attention paid to set and setting.

The basic set and setting guidelines I recommend when starting a microdosing protocol are relatively simple:

1. Don't microdose for the first time in a professional setting or if you have any professional commitments.
2. You probably won't need an experienced guide when microdosing, but some people like to have a trusted friend present.
3. Have a journal handy, perhaps some drawing or painting materials, and a plan to walk outside.

When experimenting with my own microdosing protocols, an example of an ideal combination of set and setting was when microdosing psilocybin in conjunction with therapy. The therapist knew that I was professionally involved in psychedelics, so she asked if I'd be interested in microdosing as part of our sessions after our first session. I enthusiastically agreed. By working with psilocybin in this "set and setting," it accelerated the therapeutic modality, leading to an amplified release of both sadness and anger.

Once you're comfortable with psychedelics, you might branch out with set and setting. For instance, in 2015, when I'd been using psychedelics for several years, I decided to use microdosing to become more social, engaged, and connected with my friends. So, I microdosed at a wedding, a prosocial environment full of people I knew and liked. I set my intention, chose my setting, and had a great time. Indeed, one of the most significant benefits of microdosing and minidosing is how they can help with prosociality. My microdose amplified my desire to engage at the wedding and deepened my sense of connection. However, I would never recommend microdosing at a wedding to someone just starting their psychedelic journey. The key to microdosing is to go slow and start in private settings.

Even advanced users like myself occasionally make errors. Recently, I was at a psychedelic conference in Miami and had the opportunity to sample some of the last remaining LSD from the Merry Pranksters, the infamous group led by Ken Kesey who drove a brightly painted school bus from California to New York in 1964. It was excellent acid. But I overshot it and ended up doing a little too much. The conference environment was not the best setting, and I got overwhelmed, so I did some calming nose breathing and walked around the area to center myself. Still, it wasn't ideal. Had I been less experienced, it could have been extraordinarily intense and overwhelming.

## No One-Size-Fits-All

The foundation for any individual's microdosing journey is contingent on what makes them feel psychologically safe. There is no one-size-fits-all approach. For example, whether to disclose one's microdosing to friends and family will be entirely up to the individual. If someone close to them disapproves, that could create an underlying anxiety that taints the practice. I encourage you to practice discernment in who to tell and who you interact with during your experiences. Even at lower doses, you're still more sensitive to your environment and the energy around you. Choose to be around uplifting people you can trust.

As a starting point, I recommend microdosing alone or in the presence of one trusted friend for the first four to six weeks. If you feel a significant and impactful change, you can then navigate the process of disclosing to certain people that you're microdosing. If you suspect a conversation may be difficult, emphasize the clinical research that supports the use of psychedelics. In addition, you can point to the changing legal landscape and FDA approval for clinical use. Doing some homework before entering the conversation can be a powerful way to minimize the stigma that some of your loved ones may still hold.

## Growth Mindset

It's critical to have a growth mindset before any psychedelic experience, including your microdosing protocol. The concept of "growth mindset" comes from researcher Carol Dweck, who found that people learn more effectively when they focus less on the outcome of an experience and more on enjoying the process.

Psychedelics open a space for significant change, but they aren't a magic pill. You still have to commit to change and growth to experience tangible benefits. A growth mindset sets the foundation for understanding that there's nothing inherently wrong with you. You aren't trying to fix something broken. Instead, a growth mindset allows you to anchor into a creative vision for the version of yourself that you're becoming—a robust mental frame that will help you get the most of your microdosing experience.

## Setting Intention

An intention is a conscious aim, chosen based on your values, tied to an embodied action in the future. In microdosing, your intention is your vision for who you want to be, how you want to feel, and what you might want to create. Setting a clear intention allows you to reimagine how all angles of your being contribute to your vision.

Intention always comes back to context. You must take action when the context is proper or hit the brakes when the context is wrong.

When setting your intention, try to envision what you want in clear, concrete terms. As you begin a microdosing protocol, the journey will sometimes be challenging, and your clarity of purpose will make the challenge more enjoyable and rewarding.

Your intention also creates tension between your current reality and your envisioned future. As the creator of your life, your job is to hold and utilize that tension to close the gap. And, as a final tip, always use an intention to create what you desire, not to avoid a potential negative outcome.

For example, imagine you want a healthier, more exciting, and more fulfilling relationship with your partner. However, you also realize that you've been traumatized by a loved one in the past. Knowing this, you could set an intention to release that trauma so it doesn't impact how you show up in your current relationship. A choice like this would allow you to confront the pain you feel rather than numb or deny it, so you can rewrite your story in a way that serves both your present and future self. Of course, difficult emotions may arise, but because you have the direction of your intention, you'll be willing to follow through with the process.

Let's say you think microdosing can make you more creative. Don't use "be more creative" as an intention. It's not specific or concrete. Instead, set an intention to write five chapters of a book, and look to microdosing as an accelerant to support you in that creative process. Microdosing can help you enter a flow state and minimize creative resistance as you're working on the book outline and knocking out those first five chapters.

To help this land, here are four concrete steps you can take to apply this to your own life:

## 1. Set Your Vision

Vision is your North Star. Keep it as clear, straightforward, and practical as possible. Remember, there's a difference between a life purpose and an intention. If you're feeling overwhelmed in your intention setting, try making the intention smaller and more concrete. Spend some time thinking about what matters most to you and what you want to create.

Sit for a few minutes to consider each of the following questions and write down an honest answer that comes from your heart. Don't censor yourself by worrying about what you're supposed to want or what others might think. The goal is to get as close as possible to what matters to you.

- If you could choose only one thing you could do better next month, what would it be?
- What would you like to learn more about in the next month?
- What habits would you like to improve?
  - » At work or school?
  - » With friends and family?
  - » For health?
- What type of connections would you like to make with others?
- What worthwhile and personally meaningful leisure activities would you like to pursue?

- How could you improve your relationship with your partner(s), parents, children, and/or siblings?
- What would you like to have achieved a month from now, career-wise?
- Are there specific areas in your life where you would like to gain more insight or wisdom?
- Think of someone who you admire. What qualities and virtues do they possess that you can integrate into your own life?
- What steps could you take to create a month of successfully growing toward your ideal self?
- Now, spend some time thinking about the outcome if you fail to pursue your goals and let your bad habits get out of control. What decisions would lead to a future you want to avoid?

## 2. Take Inventory

To clarify your goals for your microdosing regimen, take inventory of what changes you'd like to make in your life, focusing on the upcoming month. It can be helpful to visualize your future self, having integrated these changes into your life. Where are you in one month, and what looks different between now and your future vision?

One excellent model for this comes from *The Path of Least Resistance* by Robert Fritz. In this book, Fritz discusses the power of structural thinking and creative orientation.

He offers a relatively straightforward model to consider:

- What outcome do you want to create? Define this in a clear, visual manner.
- What is your current reality? Be as honest and objective as possible! What are the good and the not-so-good aspects?
- What are clear, executable steps to go from current reality to your envisioned future reality?

## 3. Clarify and Refine

Once you have a clear understanding of what you stand for and how you would like the upcoming month to unfold, translate your future vision into practical steps. The most potent intentions follow an "if-then" structure, also called implementation intentions. The "if" portion helps you plan for a specific moment in the future, priming you to "then" act deliberately, staying in alignment with your values.

A few examples:

- "If I get distracted from my project, then I think of why I want to complete it and return my focus to the task at hand."
- "If I feel emotionally overwhelmed, then I take a moment to breathe in and remind myself to allow any feeling to arise."

- "If I see myself judging my creative output, then I keep going because I know it doesn't need to be perfect."

Always frame your intentions in the positive. For example, "I want to trust myself" is more helpful than "I want to stop being shy." Also, be specific. Your intentions should describe a particular set of behaviors, so you will know the feeling of achieving your day's goal.

## 4. Set the Steps You Need to Take to Bring Your Vision into Reality

Microdosing can give you the courage and capacity to take the necessary steps to create your envisioned reality. Resistance to change comes from the ego because the ego likes to maintain the status quo. By minimizing your resistance to change, microdosing eases the process by which you're evolving, giving you the confidence to move forward.

After completing the above, you will ideally have a plan to bring your intention into reality. First, declare your intention: write it, speak it, record it, and internalize it. Then, hold yourself accountable for carrying out your desired actions. Each day, bring your thoughts back to your intention; these touchpoints can help guide your decisions and behavior throughout the day. You might be amazed at how smoothly you progress toward your goals.

You also might find that your outcomes aren't exactly what you envisioned, or you might change your mind about how to achieve what you want. That's not necessarily a problem. If you approach the process with integrity and honest self-reflection, you'll still mature in your awareness of who you are and what you most want to create.

## Encountering the Unexpected

When giving a public talk, I almost always microdose. Microdosing helps with articulation when presenting the material, generating more confidence while on stage. But the medicine itself isn't a magic ticket to success. I have a three-step process to ensure I get the desired results from microdosing:

1. Leading up to the talk, I prepare by writing it out, practicing it, and bouncing ideas off my advisors and friends to fine-tune it.
2. On the day of the talk, I spend time in meditation, visualizing the intention for microdosing to amplify.
3. Finally, I take the microdose.

Taking these preparatory measures helps to reduce the chances of encountering the unexpected.

In long-term microdosing protocols, the unexpected often relates to bodily experiences such as heightened emotions. Often people turn to microdosing hoping to have a light, joyful experience but end up dealing with some complicated feelings that aren't welcome. With psilocybin, I've had some heavy emotions come up, and, like I experienced in Miami, LSD can bring about some overstimulation that leads to anxiety. When dysregulated, you need to be ready to drop into some practices such as nose breathing to help regulate your responses if the unexpected occurs. Five to ten minutes of nose breathing—inhaling for a count of four and exhaling for a count of eight—will almost always bring you back to the center. Grounding is another valuable practice and can take a simple form: sitting in a comfortable chair, going to a park to walk around, or doing anything else that allows you to move a little energy and calm down.

Remember that psychedelics intensify emotions you may not be tuned into when sober. Psychedelics enhance sensitivity and bring awareness to these emotions, and we can process them by listening to them and feeling where they occur in the body.

An important effect of working with these medicines is enhanced sensitivity. The excellent news about enhanced sensitivity is that it doesn't only bring about the unexpected. It also enhances your experience of stillness and quiet, and this allows you to anchor into the calm.

### Comparing Expected Effects with Placebo

If mindset is so important, how do we know the effects of microdosing aren't due to the placebo effect?[98] To understand this question, we must first acknowledge that the mind can change our reality without the help of external substances. We have an innate, endogenous capacity to make decisions in our best interest, heal from certain diseases, and engineer the life we want to live.

In addition, research indicates that novel treatments often show greater initial efficacy when released onto the market. Often, the effectiveness of a new treatment decreases over time. There is so much hype around psychedelic research today because the results are optimistic. But there's also a sense that, over time, as more people get used to working with psychedelics, the overall efficacy will likely decrease. So, the question is: are psychedelics actually better than placebo? [99]

The answer depends on what effects we choose to measure. While I fully acknowledge the power of the placebo effect, our current metrics for microdosing remain skewed. We're examining microdosing through the same lens as macrodosing, which means looking at the tangible, physically perceptible changes—the hallucinations, somatic experiences, and emotional purging—as evidence of efficacy. If we take a very low dose and don't have visualizations, hallucinations, or significant shifts in understanding, it's easy to conclude that nothing happens. In essence, we're trying to listen to FM radio by tuning into an AM frequency.

Microdosing increases brain-derived neurotrophic factor (BDNF), a precursor to neurogenesis. Thus, the changes in our day-to-day lives through microdosing are subtle, giving us increased openness in social situations, for example, or greater creative problem-solving capacity. Therefore, I prefer to consider microdosing as a supplement, like a probiotic or vitamin that you take every day for certain health benefits.

The intention of microdosing isn't to facilitate a mystical experience but instead to see incremental changes over a longer period of time (usually thirty to sixty days). Thus, any measurement we take needs to look at the effects of microdosing over time.

What changes about certain biomarkers if I'm microdosing two or three times a week? How does it impact my sleep quality, attention span, mindfulness, and relationships? Those are the types of metrics to pay attention to when determining the effectiveness of a microdosing protocol. Unfortunately, much of the current clinical research isn't well-tuned to capture what could be exciting data about how microdosing interplays with lifestyle changes. Like anything scientific, researchers want to minimize as many variables as possible. Unfortunately, this approach overlooks the complex interconnectedness of every aspect of our lives.

## Choosing a Substance

When it comes to choosing which substance to microdose, go back to the intention of beginning your microdosing protocol. LSD tends to be more beneficial for prosociality or extroversion, like when you're in a communal environment that involves talking or social stimulation. It's lovely for hiking and being outdoors. I also love it for conversations where I explore new ideas with others.

On the other hand, psilocybin tends to be more somatic, tapping us deeper into emotions and physical sensations. People often take psilocybin in conjunction with therapy, as I did. Psilocybin helped me tune into the feelings coming up in my body and let go of certain beliefs.

For people who intend to get off pharmaceuticals, psilocybin is an attractive option because it's a natural fungus. Some people swear off synthetics entirely, including MDMA and LSD, and choose to work only with nature. Just keep in mind, not everything that nature makes is necessarily good for us. What is true, is that nature tends to bring more balance to her creations, while things made in a lab are often harvested from human evolution and have less wisdom than what the earth produces. With novel manufactured medicines, it's challenging to ascertain what potential second- or third-order consequences can be, whereas with tried-and-tested plants, we understand their effects because we've been working with them for centuries.

So, when choosing what substance to microdose with, look back at the vision you wrote down and consider the effect you'd like to create to manifest your intentions. One of the primary benefits of microdosing is that the doses are small and the results subtle. This gives you space to observe and adjust how your protocol is helping you manifest your vision.

## Want to Go Deeper?

Check out your Microdosing Mastery portal for exclusive resources, articles, and interviews to discover more about the topics from this chapter.

Just go to thethirdwave.co/bonus to access your exclusive book bonuses.

# 6

# Sourcing Psychedelics

W hile mindset matters when microdosing, sourcing the real thing—LSD or psilocybin—is the best way to ensure the safest and most reliable experience. Psychedelics themselves are not necessarily dangerous. In fact, according to neuropsychopharmacologist Dr. David Nutt, LSD and psilocybin are among the least dangerous drugs. Nevertheless, in many countries, they're still illegal.

The legal question poses an obvious problem for microdosers, as it leaves us primarily to our own devices when sourcing substances. At Third Wave, we're often asked our advice on sourcing materials for microdosing. People usually don't have an organic community from which to solicit psychedelics; they may be newcomers who have never tried them before or, if they have, they may have lost contact with their original suppliers.

In this chapter, I'll delve into some of the available options. But first, a couple of disclaimers:

- Despite the liberalization of cannabis laws (at least in the US) and the conversation around drugs in general, you may still face heavy fines and incarceration for the possession of LSD or psilocybin. The same goes for many other substances used for microdosing, including mescaline, iboga, and ayahuasca. In other words, you undertake these experiments at your own risk. Therefore, I recommend you take the necessary time to research the possible legal consequences.

- Both LSD and psilocybin have a well-documented history of safety. However, far less is known (at least scientifically) about the safety of mescaline, iboga, ayahuasca, and other psychedelics. Indeed, many of the "research chemicals" and "legal highs" (substances with slightly tweaked chemical formulas so that they're no longer illegal) often substituted for prohibited psychedelics can be risky because there is little to no record of human use. The responsibility for weighing illicit substances' potential benefits and harms is yours alone.

With that out of the way, I've endeavored to compile this chapter based on credible, up-to-date information as of mid-2022.

The legal landscape of psychedelics is changing rapidly, so please do your due diligence before embarking into this liminal space.

## Option 1: Find the Others

There's no shortage of LSD and psilocybin. And burgeoning interest in psychonautic research has fueled the supply of less known entheogens like iboga. You often just need to know the right people.

So, whenever someone asks me how to get hold of "real" substances for microdosing, I always give the same answer: start building relationships.

When I say build relationships, I don't necessarily mean with drug dealers, though that may sometimes be the case. Unfortunately, decades of ill-advised prohibitions have placed some of our most valuable and transformative tools into unsavory hands. This isn't to say that all suppliers are "drug dealers" or that all drug dealers engage in other criminal activities, but the risks and potential for ethical conflicts remain.

Fortunately, the mainstreaming of psychedelics has led to another exciting development: the resurgence of psychedelic societies. These above-ground psychedelic communities are all about forging connections and building relationships. While none of these groups supply psychedelics to members, they're all invaluable forums for building rapport and sharing experiences—not to mention integrating them.

Crucially, they're also about challenging stigma. By attracting members from wildly different backgrounds over a shared fascination with psychedelics, psychedelic societies have the potential to legitimize the field.

Here's how to get involved:

1. Do an internet search to find a psychedelic society near you.
2. Get in touch with your local society's leader.
3. Go to an event and start making connections.

These relatively casual events last two to four hours and usually include refreshments, music, and the occasional special guest. They're often well attended, as people are excited to be in a group that fully accepts them, free from stigma. There's a specific energy that comes from spending time with like-minded people and not having to hide any part of yourself. People hang out, connect, and make friends in a casual, nonjudgmental environment.

You'll get more out of this if you go in the spirit of authentic community building. However, by co-creating these networks and helping to legitimize psychedelics, you'll inevitably also come across the substances you seek.

## Option 2: Use Legal Alternatives

Depending on where you live, you may be able to find legal substitutes for both psilocybin mushrooms and LSD.

Here are some possibilities.

## Psilocybin Truffles

In the Netherlands, where psilocybin mushrooms have been illegal since 2008, it's still legal to buy psilocybin-containing truffles due to a loophole in the law.

Of course, this isn't very helpful if you don't live in the Netherlands—at least not at first glance. However, many legitimate suppliers in the Netherlands routinely ship psilocybin truffles abroad. And even in the UK, where nonmedical "psychoactive substances" are uniformly banned, authorities consider such imports a relatively low priority for law enforcement.

While buying truffles online is still a punishable crime in most countries and not without risk, it's an attractive option for many.

Alternatively, if you live in one of the Schengen Area countries, especially if you're close to the Netherlands, you could feasibly buy truffles in person and return home overland to avoid the risk of detection.

## 4-ACO-DMT

4-ACO-DMT is a synthetic tryptamine with structural similarities to psilocybin and psilocin. Doses as low as two to 3 mg can increase empathy and introspection, lift dark moods, and enhance visual perception. While some find microdoses a little too sedating for productivity at work, others find 4-ACO-DMT makes them more alert.

Either way, you're free to experiment for yourself, unless you live in the UK, Italy, Sweden, Belgium, or Brazil where this substance is banned.

## 1P-LSD

1P-LSD (1-propionyl-lysergic acid diethylamide) is a semi-synthetic analog of LSD. In other words, it's closely related both structurally and chemically to lysergic acid diethylamide. According to some, it may only differ in absorption rate, duration, metabolism, and excretion. It may even be a "prodrug," converted to LSD by the body. Little is known for sure, but the effects of 1P-LSD are remarkably close to its relative.

For now, at least, it's legal to buy in most European countries, the US, and Canada. If caught with it in some countries, including the US (although it's not federally scheduled), authorities may view 1P-LSD as an (illegal) analog of an illicit substance. But it's widely available online.

## Other LSD Analogs

Numerous other "research chemical" analogs of LSD offer comparable dosage and effect profiles. They include AL-LAD, ALD-52, ETH-LAD, PRO-LAD, and LSZ.

Anecdotal reports list alertness, clarity, mood enhancement, and cognitive elasticity among their effects when microdosed. Some users even prefer these analogs to LSD.

In some countries, however, their legal status is unclear. For example, as with 1P-LSD, possession in the US may or may not be prosecuted under the Federal Analogue Act; the law itself is ambiguously worded, and case law is limited.[100] They also tend to be illegal in countries that take a more proactively suppressive approach to new drugs, including the UK, Latvia, Sweden, and Switzerland.

## Ergoloid Mesylates (Hydergine)

Developed by Albert Hofmann and marketed without FDA approval as a neuroprotective "smart drug," a regular dose of ergoloid mesylates as labeled feels qualitatively like a microdose of LSD.

It's only available on prescription in most Western countries, but you may be able to buy it online elsewhere.

## 2C-B-FLY

Even at sub-milligram doses, the effects of 2C-B-FLY feel like mescaline and MDA (MDMA's more potent, more psychedelic predecessor). Microdoses of less than 100 μg (0.1 mg) may enhance motivation, empathy, creativity, and philosophical or abstract thinking.

2C-B-FLY is unscheduled in the US but may be considered an illegal analog of 2C-B. In Canada, it's a Schedule III substance.

In any case, it's widely available online.

## Amanita Muscaria

Amanita muscaria—also known as the fly agaric mushroom—is entirely legal in most countries. Notable exceptions include Australia, the Netherlands, and the UK.

Amanitas contain muscimol and ibotenic acid (not psilocybin and psilocin), so their effects differ from traditional psilocybin mushrooms. Microdoses of 0.1 to 0.5 g can relieve anxiety, enhance mood, increase energy, and generally impart a sense of "magic" to the world through insights and synchronicities.

## Option 3: Grow Your Own

LSD is too complex (and legally risky) for most people to synthesize at home. But other substances for microdosing are relatively easy to cultivate.

### Psilocybin

Although psilocybin mushrooms remain illegal in most countries, spores are often legal. That means you can start growing your own for a consistent private supply. Home cultivation also minimizes the risk of misidentifying mushrooms in the wild.

Finding the medicine is the biggest challenge people face when starting to microdose. We address that by empowering people to grow their own medicine. Third Wave offers a kit that makes it easy to grow mushrooms at home.[101] We also have a course on using the grow kit, with additional educational materials. We do not include spores, though you can source them legally in every state except Georgia, Idaho, and California. Spores are easy to find, and we offer guidance on buying spores on the Third Wave website.

## Ergine (LSA)

Ergine, or lysergic acid amide (LSA), is similar to LSD with vaguely comparable effects. Users tend to find it more sedating, nauseating, and generally less potent than LSD. However, microdoses can boost mental clarity and focus while relieving anxiety and depression.

It's also naturally occurring, and while the compound itself is widely illegal, ergine-containing seeds are not. Morning glories and Hawaiian baby woodrose are among the best-known plant sources. Both are legal to grow in the US (except Arizona), the UK, and mainland Europe (except Italy).

Common microdoses fall in the range of five to fifteen morning glory seeds or 0.33 to 3 Hawaiian baby woodrose seeds. Usually, they're chewed for about twenty minutes and held under the tongue to absorb the ergine sublingually.

## Mescaline

Cacti are well known as some of the easiest plants to grow, practically taking care of themselves given the right conditions. And mescaline-containing cacti, such as peyote and San Pedro, are legal in most countries.

In the US, only members of the Native American Church can legally cultivate peyote. However, San Pedro can freely be grown for ornamental purposes.

## Ibogaine

Iboga, including the whole plant and seeds, is illegal in the US. Many European countries also restrict it, and Australia and Canada, but seeds are widely available for shipping elsewhere.

Although adapted for the humid conditions of West African rainforests, iboga can adjust to drier climates as long as temperatures remain well above 59°F.

## Ayahuasca

Plants used in traditional ayahuasca brews—including Banisteriopsis caapi and Psychotria viridis—are also adapted for the rainforest, so they need plenty of heat and moisture. As a result, they may need to be grown indoors. They can also take months or years to mature.

B. caapi delivers MAOIs and is used to ensure that the body does not break down DMT before it crosses the blood-brain barrier. Both plants are legal in many countries, even if their alkaloids are not. But there are plenty of alternatives. These include Syrian rue, passionflower, and yohimbe for the MAOIs; and Mimosa hostilis, chaliponga, and reed canary grass for the DMT.

## Protecting Your Identity

Keep in mind that nothing can truly guarantee your anonymity online. Proxy networks and cryptocurrencies are the only ways to mitigate the risk. However, assuming your seller is genuine, law enforcement could still hack them.

In June 2017, for instance, Dutch authorities seized Hansa, one of the largest darknet marketplaces. However, instead of shutting it down, they continued to run it as usual, secretly collecting user data and transaction details. Meanwhile, the FBI shut down AlphaBay, another central marketplace, to funnel its users toward Hansa. Ultimately, Europol gathered ten thousand postal addresses and made numerous arrests.

While it's true that the government is becoming less and less interested in cracking down on psychedelic use, it's still in your best interest to take a few measures to ensure you're operating safely.

It's helpful to have a basic level of proficiency in Bitcoin or other cryptocurrencies. Cryptocurrency transactions are more secure and private than your typical fiat currency transaction and, therefore, often used in sourcing methodology. Decentralized finance is the way to maneuver around things like banks blocking credit card transactions, which was common in the early days of the cannabis industry. Consider downloading an encrypted messaging app such as Signal, owned by a nonprofit, whereas Meta owns WhatsApp. Always be aware of whom you're giving your information and data to.

These general privacy practices are good disciplines to cultivate whether or not you're working with psychedelics. If you aren't dealing a ton of LSD or mushrooms, chances are, no one is going to come after you. So, it's essential to strike a balance. Don't let the fear of being caught stop you from engaging with these helpful medicines, and at the same time, practice some general privacy measures to stay under the radar.

Whichever route you choose, stay safe.

## Want to Go Deeper?

Check out your Microdosing Mastery portal for exclusive resources, articles, and interviews to discover more about the topics from this chapter.

Just go to thethirdwave.co/bonus to access your exclusive book bonuses.

# 7

# Preparing Your Microdose

S o, you've sourced your preferred psychedelic substance, and now you're eager to start microdosing. But before we go deep into the world of microdosing protocol, let's first cover the basics on how to properly prepare your medicine.

## Preparing LSD Microdoses

### Paper Tabs

The most well-known preparation method for LSD is the paper tab (also known as a blotter). The tab of LSD is often cut up and then taken in tiny pieces. Although cutting up the tab is a common method, it's far from ideal for several reasons:

### Reason #1: LSD Concentration May Be Uneven

During manufacturing, blotter sheets of individual tabs are soaked in a liquid LSD solution and dried. However, this drying process is sometimes uneven. As a result, some paper parts are more concentrated than others. Because we're so sensitive to the molecule—and because we use such small amounts for microdosing—even the tiniest variations in potency can make all the difference.

### Reason #2: Tabs Are Minuscule

The standard size is a quarter inch squared, so you might struggle to cut ten or more equal pieces out of a normal sized tab.

### Reason #3: You Risk Wasting the Chemical

The longer you spend handling tabs, exposing them to light, air, and heat—as well as moisture if you're not wearing gloves—the more likely you are to degrade your LSD.

In short, cutting up tabs isn't worth the hassle, especially when a far more effective and much more manageable method is available.

## Volumetric Microdosing

Volumetric microdosing ensures consistency by dissolving your tab's LSD content in a sterile liquid solution. It would help if you had a small bottle, a one ml syringe (with a blunt needle), and some distilled water or vodka.

Follow these steps to get started:

## 1. Prepare Your Container

If you have a dark glass bottle or something opaque for your solution, make sure the inside is sanitized. If your bottle is clear, on the other hand, you will need to sanitize the container and shield its contents from light damage. Tinfoil works fine.

## 2. Fill It with Vodka or Distilled Water

For a standard 100-microgram (μg) tab, use ten ml of solvent—either distilled water, vodka, or both. This way, one ml of your solution will contain precisely 10 μg of LSD, and you can reliably adjust this dose up and down by the graduations on your syringe.

Alternatively, you may use a shop-bought miniature (fifty ml) bottle of vodka. Of course, you'll need to consume more alcohol for the same dose, but it won't be enough to get tipsy.

If you choose to use water, make sure you use distilled water! The chlorine in tap water destroys LSD upon contact. For this reason, you should also avoid consuming chlorinated water, or brushing your teeth with it, for at least one hour before and after you microdose.

## 3. Add LSD

Drop one tab of acid into your vodka or water and secure the lid. Then shake it and store it in a cool, dark place. A fridge is ideal, but you'll probably want to label the bottle if the fridge is shared. Otherwise, anywhere out of heat and light is fine. Leave the solution for twenty-four hours or so before you use it. The tab won't dissolve, but it's OK to leave it in the bottle if you've used vodka. If you've used distilled water, though, you should fish it out with tweezers to minimize the risk of contamination.

Your solution should last at least a few months and probably longer if you've used vodka.

## 4. Measure Your First Microdose

It helps to know the dose on your tabs, but that's not always possible. So, if you don't know for sure, assume that each tab contains 100 μg of acid. Then, divide this number by the volume (ml) of your solution to calculate how many micrograms of LSD are in each milliliter.

The standard microdose falls between 10 and 20 μg, so if you have ten ml of solution, you'll need between one and two (one ml) syringes' worth for a dose. If you've used fifty ml, you'll need five to ten syringes' worth for a dose (or a bigger syringe!).

## Preparing Psilocybin Microdoses

As with LSD, it's tempting to cut up psilocybin mushrooms and take little bits as your microdoses. Again, however, this won't ensure you're taking consistent amounts of medicine. Psilocybin concentration differs between strains, between individual mushrooms within the same strain, and even between the caps and stems of the same mushrooms. In addition, the potency often depends more on maturity and growing conditions than on size.

Surprisingly, immature "pins" may contain more psilocybin than older, fully grown mushrooms.

The best way to ensure a consistent microdose is to choose a strain and stick to it. It's OK to experiment, but you may have to start with a low-end microdose each time you try a new strain. It's much easier and more reliable to pick a strain and keep it.

Here's how to prepare psilocybin:

## 1. Dry Your Mushrooms

There are several different methods for drying mushrooms, ranging in price and efficiency. The quickest and most dependable—but also the most expensive—method is to use a food dehydrator, available for about forty dollars. Using a dehydrator will get your mushrooms "cracker dry." They'll snap when you try to bend them, which is exactly the consistency you want for grinding. You can also air-dry your mushrooms with a fan and then place them in an airtight container. It takes longer but is both cheap and efficient.

## 2. Grind Them Up

You'll need a set of digital scales (accurate to at least 0.1 g, or 100 mg) and a coffee grinder.

Weigh out enough of your dried mushrooms for the amount and size of the microdoses you want to prepare. On average, microdoses range between 200 to 500 mg. So, if you're new to microdosing, especially if you're new to psilocybin, you may want to start with four grams for twenty microdoses of 200 mg each. Then, of course, you can always increase your dose by taking more as you go along.

Next, place your dried mushrooms into a coffee grinder and pulse for up to a minute. Be sure to allow time for the particles to settle since if you open the chamber too soon, you may lose a lot of the powder. It's also advisable to use a different coffee grinder than the one you usually use for your coffee, as the blades can be hard to clean. I'm assuming you don't want psychedelic residue in your coffee—not least because of the earthy taste.

Using a coffee grinder should result in a fine powder with an even distribution of psilocybin, and this is perfect for microdosing.

## 3. Transfer the Powder for Storage

Many people use a capsule machine or homemade tamping rod to transfer the powder to capsules. If you go this route, start with the "Size 3" capsules since each one holds about 200 mg depending on how you pack them.

Alternatively, you could transfer all your powder to a Mason jar for storage and weigh out as much as you need each time you want a microdose, adding it to juice, honey, or cereal as desired. The downside to this method? Repeated exposure to air and potential condensation whenever you open the jar. But you should be all right if you don't grind too much at a time. Prepare enough for a couple of weeks at most.

Whichever method you choose, psilocybin will last the longest in the freezer. Just make sure it's in an airtight container, ideally with a silica gel packet.

## Preparing Iboga Microdoses

When microdosing iboga, many people consume the root bark. One gram appears to be a good starting point. An alternative method is to grind it and fill capsules with 500 mg each.

As with LSD and psilocybin, however, the concentration of the primary psychoactive compound (in this case, ibogaine) varies. Extracts are therefore widely preferred, not only for consistency but also to get the most bang for your buck.

Although illegal in several countries, including the US (but curiously not the UK), most individuals can purchase iboga extracts online. Most users prefer the concentrated total alkaloid (TA) tincture, of which just one drop is usually enough for a microdose. The TA extract is also available in powder form. You may need 50 to 100 mg of this, which you can swallow in a capsule or stir into liquid.

Alternatively, you may wish to start with a 25 mg dose of an isolated ibogaine HCl extract. Some say it offers a shallower experience, but it's a purer form of the primary psychoactive alkaloid.

## Preparing Mescaline Microdoses

Mescaline, like ibogaine, is one of the many alkaloids present in peyote, torch cactus, San Pedro, and several other psychoactive cacti. Like psilocybin mushrooms, the concentrations vary across species. If you can't find extracted mescaline and don't want to extract it yourself, eating the raw material is acceptable.[102] Various Native American groups are known to "microdose" peyote while hunting to improve their stamina. However, if you choose to microdose with mescaline, we recommend working with San Pedro. Unfortunately, peyote is an endangered species, while San Pedro grows plentifully in many parts of the US.

## Step 1: Acquire or Grow San Pedro Cactus

San Pedro cacti are legal and easy to obtain and grow. You can buy them at most home improvement stores such as Home Depot. San Pedro also grows from cuttings, and many people get their first cactus by receiving a cutting from a friend. We have an extensive blog about the care and cultivation of San Pedro on the Third Wave website, which will give you a much more in-depth look at this cactus if you're interested.[103]

## Step 2: Harvest and Dry the Cactus

Once the cactus is ready for harvest, cut it into chunks. Dry the pieces in the sun, oven, or food dehydrator. Grind the dried chunks into powder. Ingesting the powder gives you the full spectrum of the cactus's alkaloids and the mescaline. It's a good idea to put the powder into gelatin capsules to swallow, as the taste of San Pedro cactus is revolting.

Take some time to experiment for yourself to find the correct dosage. The amount needed varies from person to person, but a single microdose can typically range from 10 to 20 grams of fresh San Pedro (a one- or two-inch slice) or 3.5 to 10 grams of dried San Pedro.

## Want to Go Deeper?

Check out your Microdosing Mastery portal for exclusive resources, articles, and interviews to discover more about the topics from this chapter.

Just go to thethirdwave.co/bonus to access your exclusive book bonuses.

# 8

# Microdosing Protocols

As microdosers, we're also pioneers. Any person who chooses to commit to a microdosing protocol goes courageously into the unknown, playing with trial and error, to land on what is ideal for their context and specific situation. When beginning your microdosing journey, procedural constraints (protocols), can help to guide you in established best practices, maximizing the initial benefits and mitigating potential downside and risk.

## The Fadiman Protocol

One of the most popular microdosing protocols follows Dr. Fadiman's sequence, which was built by collecting early reports from self-study participants. Fadiman designed his research protocol primarily to collect meaningful (i.e., standardized) data from a large sample, deliberately returning participants to baseline consciousness as an experimental control.

The routine is to take one microdose in the morning on day one and day four of each week. So, if you take your first microdose on a Sunday, you'll take your second on a Wednesday, spending the other days of the week reflecting upon and observing the residual effects.[104]

Throughout each cycle, you should keep notes on the effects of each dose—things like your mental state, emotions, behavior, and so on—while following your everyday routine. Journaling helps to keep tabs on your feelings and cultivates awareness of your present state. Even at higher doses, a huge part of successful integration is anchoring into the emotions you experience. Journaling is an effective tool in your toolkit to help you understand your relationship with the substances. When reflecting on your experiences, you can flip back into your notes and notice how different doses affected you.

Fadiman recommends an initial term of ten microdosing days, spread out over five weeks. Once you pause taking the substance, you'll have a chance to gauge how you've been affected. After the initial protocol, some people stop microdosing completely, and others, more commonly, continue to microdose on an ad hoc basis. If you microdose for a while and notice the benefits, you may be tempted to microdose daily.

Which brings up an important question: is it safe to microdose every single day? Because we don't yet know enough about the long-term effects of microdosing, it might not be wise to jump from the initial protocol straight into more cycles, although many do. Paul Stamets, for example, recommends repeated multi-day dosing, as we'll see next.

## The Paul Stamets Protocol

Paul Stamets is the world's leading authority on the medicinal and environmental use of mushrooms, including psilocybin mushrooms.

In November 2017, Paul appeared on the Joe Rogan podcast, where he spoke about a slightly different protocol than Dr. Fadiman's.

Whereas Fadiman recommends his twice-per-week protocol—one day on two days off—Stamets suggests four days on and three days off. Further, Stamets recommends combining the microdose with other medicinal mushrooms for synergistic benefits. The "Stamets Stack" combines psilocybin with lion's mane and niacin. Under this protocol, the microdoser takes about 100 milligrams of psilocybin, 500 to 1000 milligrams of lion's mane, and 50 to 200 milligrams of niacin. Stamets hypothesized the benefits of this nootropic stack, saying, "This unique combination of compounds can be incorporated into other therapies with such combination providing unique advantages for medically significant advancements, repairing neurons, removing amyloid plaques, improving mental health cognition, agility, and improving overall ecology of consciousness."[105]

Stamets believes that psilocybin will continue to help humans evolve by raising the level of global consciousness. In addition, several studies have shown that psilocybin extends the fear response, thus creating new neurological pathways when faced with a threatening situation.

Stamets also believes that microdosing's efficacy in epigenetic neurogenesis has the potential to initiate the next quantum leap in human consciousness. Such a belief plays off the Stoned Ape Theory, initially proposed by Dennis and Terence McKenna in 1992. The McKennas suggested that in small doses, psychedelic compounds increased visual acuity, making ancient users better hunters, resulting in more food, a higher reproduction rate, and greater social bonding that diversified the gene pool. Their theory supposedly helped to explain the rapid doubling in size of the human brain, which occurred in as little as 200,000 years.

In short, Stamets treats microdosing more like an ongoing supplement regimen intended to consistently strengthen connectivity between neurological nodes. In contrast, Fadiman treats microdosing as a short-term intervention to help get people "unstuck" from specific medical conditions. Your intention for microdosing will inform which protocol you choose to utilize.

## Tolerance: To Continue or Not?

Tolerance happens when, over time, the user requires higher doses of a substance to achieve the original effect. Psychedelics behave differently from many other drugs in that users seem to build up little to no tolerance to the drug with long-term use. For that reason, tolerance is a nonstarter as long as there's a forty-eight-hour window between each dose.

Currently, we know less about tolerance as it applies to microdosing than we do high doses. Each protocol outlined above is still somewhat experimental. As an example, Fadiman pays more attention to tolerance in his protocol than Stamets. Experiences vary widely between individuals.

Additionally, some people appear to be more sensitive than others. Many people microdose daily and report no tolerance effect whatsoever. Others find the effects diminish with regular use. Still, others say that the best way to benefit from microdosing is to space each dose two weeks apart!

When planning your schedule, keep in mind that the effects of psychedelics linger after the original experience. As Fadiman points out, the residual effects of LSD at standard doses last weeks, not just the twelve or so hours of the trip itself. Similarly, the residual effects of microdosing can last up to two days. That means using it daily may be an unnecessary waste of your supply.[106]

## Third Wave Protocol: Intuitive Dosing

Third Wave's protocol balances those of Fadiman and Stamets and extends beyond them into a concept called "intuitive microdosing." However, Third Wave's protocol is better for "advanced users," those who have already made it through their first microdosing protocol and wish to deepen their overall skillset.

Once you feel like you've hit a certain degree of mastery with microdosing, you can make small, iterative changes while using it and intuitively adapt your protocol to your own life, body, and goals.

Third Wave's approach focuses less on the days-on/days-off model and more on *mastering* microdosing. To master means to intuitively know the range of experiences that are possible, and thus to choose a specific amount that will support your intentions for any particular day.

Imagine you've completed one of the fundamental protocols, journaled thoroughly, and then stepped away for a few weeks of reflection. You wake up one morning on a day when you have some creative work ahead of you, or perhaps a coaching session, or even something as simple as a hike with a friend. You've noticed in your time away from microdosing that you've felt down and without much energy. You also know from your previous experience that LSD improves your mood. So, on this particular day, because your schedule is flexible and free, you decide to take twenty micrograms of LSD—which is on the high end of a microdose—rather than your typical dose of ten micrograms. You choose this dose because you intuitively know that this amount previously helped you get into flow, boosted your mood, or dropped you into deep connection with nature.

So, imagine what might be possible with thirty micrograms of LSD? Or fifty micrograms of LSD? Imagine how you may want to use 100 mg or 500 mg of psilocybin. Once you can intuitively calibrate your dose to your intention for the day, a certain level of manifestation mastery becomes available to you.

Intuitive microdosing means cultivating and developing a relationship with these substances at varying amounts, thereby understanding which dose levels support which intentions.

## Specialized Protocols

Fadiman's basic protocol is an ideal framework for starting. But depending on your specific reasons for microdosing (see Chapter 5 on intentions), you may wish to add further, more specialized protocols that better serve your aims. To this end, we've developed several suggestions.

### For Acute Anxiety

As discussed, microdosing helps people to ease their anxiety. Others, however, have found that microdosing increases anxiety. In many cases, you can adjust the timing of your doses to prevent this kind of issue.

Timing matters because microdosing, particularly with LSD, can disrupt your sleeping patterns with its relatively long duration. If you've ever suffered from anxiety, you'll know the importance of getting the right amount of sleep.

You may be able to preserve your sleep cycle by microdosing as early in the day as possible—ideally before 10:00 a.m. Generally, it would help if you aimed to microdose at least twelve hours before bed.

If you find that microdosing seems to increase your anxiety, as some do, you may want to try the following:

- Remember that psychedelics often increase patience and compassion toward others and toward self. Observe these traits above all others and reinforce them through journaling, which strengthens and promotes the developing neural pathways that underpin them.
- Use deep breathing exercises to detach yourself physically from anxious thoughts.[107] "Box breathing" is a good example. Breathe in for a count of four, hold in for four, breathe out for four, hold out for four, and start the process again for four repetitions.
- Integrate meditation and regular exercise into your microdosing protocol.
- Spend time in nature and away from modern technology. Make this a regular part of your routine.

## For Generalized Anxiety Disorder

Anxiety isn't always manageable with lifestyle adjustments. It can be extremely persistent, manifesting without identifiable cause as a generalized anxiety disorder. In this case, according to Fadiman and Korb's research, microdosing could potentially exacerbate anxiety symptoms.

Interestingly, generalized anxiety may worsen not because the drug is directly causing symptoms but because it increases your awareness of the underlying causes. That experience is seldom comfortable, but microdosing may allow you to work through your blind spots and organize yourself and your surroundings to better support you. That's why I don't mean to imply that you should avoid it altogether. Just proceed with caution, preparing for subconscious issues to surface.

Of course, if you do feel that microdosing worsens your symptoms without doing anything to help them in the long-term, you should probably lower your dose or stop consuming psychedelics entirely. Microdosing isn't for everyone, at least not right away. You may want to return to it later, perhaps after more success in treating your generalized anxiety disorder with other approaches like meditation, exercise, and prioritizing quality sleep.

## For Social Anxiety

If you experience social anxiety, on the other hand, microdosing holds much promise. In almost all cases, social anxiety responds positively to microdosing. For example, I have heard reports from many folks enthused about feeling less "in their head" and more "in the moment" when microdosing. This effect is crucial for turning down the volume on the fear of negative judgment that may be swirling around in your head and preventing you from interacting with others.

Still, you may want to take things slowly at first. For example, you could start by microdosing around the people you're closest to, then, as an experimental protocol, expand to other situations you found uncomfortable before.

## For Depression

According to anecdotal reports, microdosing works wonders for depression, as we have discussed. However, it's best not to think of it as a magic pill but as an aid to doing the hard work of healing from depression.

For all the relief people find in microdosing, many fall into old, depressive mindsets after they stop. That's why it's crucial to spend your microdosing time making positive changes to outlast the protocol itself.

For example, you may adopt new habits that support your mental health, including better nutrition, regular meditation, and exercise. You could also set aside some time each day to think about what you're grateful for. It might sound hokey, but research supports the benefits of practicing inward gratitude.[108]

## For ADD/ADHD

If you're microdosing to replace ADD/ADHD medications like Adderall, Vyvanse, or Ritalin, expect the effects to be subtler and the benefits to incrementally develop through intentional use.

For instance, if you tend to be self-critical, like many with ADD/ADHD, journaling while microdosing can help. Recording changes in your self-image can help to strengthen and reinforce new perspectives as they develop.

Remember that you will need to stop taking your conventional ADD/ADHD medications during the microdosing protocol. We do not advise microdosing psychedelics during your regular course of treatment as the increased heart strain and mental "speediness" may detract from the benefits and harm your health. On the other hand, stopping your medications suddenly may also be problematic. So, first, wean off slowly (with the support of a medical professional, always). And then, once you've weaned off, give microdosing a try.

For people with ADD/ADHD impulsivity, it's helpful to decide to refrain from making significant decisions before attempting a microdosing protocol. Microdosing amplifies impulsivity, so it's wise to be wary of the synergistic impact of combining already impulsive proclivities with this powerful tool.

## For Personal Growth

Of course, you might not be looking to "solve" anything by microdosing. Instead, you may be curious how the practice deepens your personal development and growth. If this is the case, you're likely to benefit from extended breaks between each run of ten cycles, at least if you plan to repeat the protocol. That way, you don't become psychologically dependent on microdosing.

One central tenet of any personal development program— microdosing or not—is clarifying your intention and getting clear on the outcome you desire. To ensure accelerated evolution through microdosing, set significant time aside before beginning a protocol to think through a few questions:

- If you could choose only one thing to do better next month, what would you choose?
- What type of connections would you like to make with others?
- Think of someone who you admire. What qualities and virtues do they possess that you would like to practice this month?

Sometimes, even with journaling and internal inquiry, we don't fully understand all the changes microdosing inspires and how they may be linked. I encourage you to ask trusted friends and family for feedback. If you have a spouse or partner or spend significant time with a group of friends, ask them to comment on changes they notice while you're microdosing. Examples include less reactivity when in conflict; better mood; increased energy; increased general optimism, compassion, openness, and sociability; and increased presence and awareness.

Integrate positive and constructive feedback when reflecting on how microdosing has helped accelerate your path of personal development.

## For Creativity

If you're specifically interested in microdosing for creativity, you might like to try a slightly higher dose—a mini or "museum" dose.

A "museum" dose is the amount you would take if you were going to an art museum or a concert and wanted to amplify your sensual experience without tripping. With a museum dose, you're still going to navigate life well, and you'll appreciate beautiful things even more without having any visual changes or hallucinations. A museum dose of LSD would be anywhere from thirty-five to fifty micrograms. For psilocybin, it could be anywhere from a half gram to a gram.

Unlike microdosing, minidosing is slightly perceptible. For example, if microdosing LSD is approximately fifteen micrograms for you, then a minidose may be closer to twenty-five to thirty micrograms.

The higher the dose, the more divergent—abstract and nonlinear —your thinking can become, which is the essence of creativity.

The goal is to reach a level of divergent thinking that supports creativity without moving into territory where your thinking becomes so divergent that you lose the ability or will to *create*. Mini or museum doses fall between a microdose and a full trip and strike this agreeable balance.

A critical note about facilitating creative insight with microdosing: it is vital not to rely solely on psychedelic substances to engender creative insight. As I've emphasized throughout this book, the environment in which you micro or minidose is just as important as the substance itself.

If micro or minidosing for creative purposes, I've found two techniques to be most helpful:

1. Spending time in nature with close friends and/or business partners
2. Spending time alone with a journal and pen and letting your mind wander (i.e., brainstorming on psychedelics)

These techniques minimize distractions and create a space to let your mind wander, delving deep into conceptualization and amplifying the creative process in a myriad of ways.

## For Leadership

Many have found microdosing to be an excellent tool for developing modern leadership skills. We'll look more closely at this in Chapter 12, but it's crucial to observe your behavior and how people react to you if this is your focus.

As previously mentioned, it is important to be wary and mindful of impulsivity. Implement protocols that ensure responsible decision-making, such as postponing decisions until the second day after a microdose.

Above all, keep in mind that your role as a leader is to nurture, not dominate, others. The idea is to attract people to your vision, not coerce them into it. Try to cultivate a strong habit of reflexivity in your journaling and day-to-day interactions.

## Indigenous Protocols

Much of this chapter applies to virtually any substance for micro-dosing, but some people also devise protocols for using specific plant medicines. These indigenous protocols approach psychedelic substances with respect and reverence, either as spiritual sacraments or as beings in their own right, calling to mind the Bwiti reverence of iboga, the Quechua concept of ayahuasca (meaning "spirit vine"), and the Huichol deification of peyote.

Iboga is a trusted tool for deep healing among the Bwiti people in Gabon and Cameroon. Higher doses bring insight, awareness, and deep spiritual cleansing. Smaller amounts are also considered powerful healing tools. Many people associate hospitals with death in Ghana, so visiting an herbalist or a local healer is common. These local healers and herbalists will often use small amounts of iboga as part of their toolkits. Stories and anthropological evidence point to the native use of small amounts of iboga to help with sharper vision, hunting, and other performance enhancements.

In places like the Sacred Valley and the high Andes in South America, small doses of *huachuma* (San Pedro) are used as a performance tool to help with hiking, navigating the mountains, and sustained energy. In addition, microdosing is used to heal sickness, similar to how we in the Western world use antibiotics, ibuprofen, or Tylenol. The main difference is that even at small doses, indigenous use is marked by an appreciation for the medicine's ability to nourish the soul, lift the spirit, and reconnect to nature.

Ayahuasca is used similarly by indigenous people. Sometimes, small doses are given to children from a young age so by the time they're grown, they have a strong relationship with it. Shamans or curanderos also use it in rituals to work their culture's magic. While ayahuasca is often used in beautiful and traditional ways, it sometimes falls into the wrong hands and is used for purposes of "dark magic." Further, complex admixtures happen, where shamans will mix ayahuasca with plants like belladonna, toé, or tobacco. Such potions can be highly risky and are often used for nefarious purposes.

Magic can also happen in microforms. Often, a small amount taken with an intention produces an unseen alchemy that leads to synchronicity, intuitive downloads, and an equanimous ease by which life unfolds. Unfortunately, modern microdosing substances often come in pill form, which lends itself to being a more transactional experience rather than an intuitive one. Such a frame emphasizes practical usage that is at odds with the indigenous worldview of connecting to the more profound spirit of medicine and the support it offers.

The better we know specific medicines, the more refined our approach becomes in that realm of "magic" because magic is about bending the laws of reality. It's about manifesting things previously thought to be impossible. It's about tapping into something that the rational, linear mind can't quite process.

Devising rituals based on traditional concepts, particularly if such imagery moves you, could potentiate the effects. One ibogaine microdoser, for example, recommends "letting in the spirit of iboga" to manifest positive affirmations and intentions like "I am complete," "This day is perfect," "Life is generous," or "My body is healing itself."[109]

Because these indigenous medicines carry cultural significance, I urge those who want to work with them to do so under the supervision or guidance of an indigenous elder or practitioner familiar with the medicine. In addition, experimenting with indigenous medicines requires more intentionality beyond the basic protocols I have explained for microdosing LSD or psilocybin.

You can learn more about plant medicines and their cultural significance from Third Wave's website and various other sources to research and refine your own magical protocols. It is important to cultivate a healthy respect for these powerful medicines and their histories to not only build a positive relationship with them but to safely benefit from them as well.

## Build a Relationship

The frame from which we approach intuitive dosing assumes a relationship between you and the medicine. So, first, you need to understand which dose amounts facilitate which experiences and how the medicine impacts you. Then, once this relationship is in place, you will ask: "What do I want to create with my day, and how can a microdose support me in that creation?" Other versions of this question are:

- What do I want to explore?
- What do I want to process?
- What do I want to reveal?
- What do I want to be inspired by?

There are many ways to frame a day, whether it calls for inspiration, creative brainstorming, expansion, or even intense physical demands.

Intuitive dosing requires patience, mindful practice, and clear intentions. Then we can listen to ourselves and do what's best in each moment.

## Want to Go Deeper?

Check out your Microdosing Mastery portal for exclusive resources, articles, and interviews to discover more about the topics from this chapter.

Just go to thethirdwave.co/bonus to access your exclusive book bonuses.

# 9

# Reflecting on and Refining Your Protocol

Whatever your goals for microdosing and whichever protocol you choose, you will eventually finish your initial experiment. Do you continue or not? What is the best way to proceed if you decide to go on? How soon do you start your next microdosing protocol?

After finishing my first microdosing protocol in January 2016, I found myself at a crossroads. This initial protocol lasted for seven months at a pace of two times per week. And I didn't really want to stop. My experiment had gone off without a hitch: creative projects flourished, my confidence and charisma skyrocketed in social situations, and complex thoughts and ideas became easy to articulate in a clear and meaningful manner. Unfortunately, I had plans to leave Thailand and travel to Taiwan, and I preferred to minimize my risk by not carrying an illicit substance with me. So, I stopped.

I also had other reservations. While I felt a deep sense of contentment with the level of transformation from microdosing and had yet to experience any negative consequences, I did not want to become psychologically dependent on an external substance for engendering change. I also didn't know enough about the risks of consistently taking low amounts of LSD over an extended period.

I needed to find a middle ground. That meant experimenting with different intervals of microdosing in between protocols. But, more crucially, it meant taking time to get back to baseline and explore what had changed about my inner world since starting that initial microdosing protocol.

If you find yourself in a similar place, I suggest digging back through your old notes to take an honest, critical look at how you've developed. Ask yourself questions like:

- Have I achieved the goals I set out to (or have my priorities shifted)?
- Am I approaching my work, relationships, health, and other areas of my life any differently?
- Has my self-image changed?
- How do I feel about the future?
- What about the past?
- Have I learned anything else?

When applying this to my own life, I looked back at notes from May 2015 when I'd just begun microdosing. I'd recently started my first entrepreneurial project and was barely making ends meet. Still, I was very driven and motivated in my work and equally dedicated to creating more freedom for myself.

When I started microdosing, I had two core intentions: first, to spend more time in flow, reducing creative resistance with the intent of building a bigger business to reach more people; and second, to reduce my social anxiety and my reliance on alcohol in social situations, and to remain present when out of my comfort zone.

Doing this work was fundamental to how I now live my life. I created an awareness that allowed me to build a foundation from which, now, six years later, I can support myself, work from anywhere, work any hours I want, and be free to express myself.

Being exposed to microdosing was powerful in and of itself. I learned a new modality that had the capacity to create positive change. On top of that, I dove into the history of psychedelics to better understand why these powerful, profound substances remain illegal today. I learned as much as I could about the topic, and, since then, have started multiple companies to educate people about psychedelics. If I'd never begun microdosing, it's unlikely that I would've followed that path.

My relationship with microdosing LSD and psilocybin taught me a lot about the autonomy and agency I can have if I live in a sense of truth and power. Through intentional psychedelic use, I remind myself of my capacity to create.

As you reflect on your own experiences, the final question—whether you learned anything else (for example, about yourself, others, or life in general)—may be the most important. Microdosing can have surprising personal outcomes, shining a light on previously hidden parts of your psyche. Ultimately, by taking time away from it, you'll be able to identify clear, practical foci for future cycles.

It may be helpful to go over all these points with somebody who knows you well, especially regarding relationship inquiries. For example, you might talk with a significant other, a close friend, or a therapist. Ideally, they'll have seen you frequently throughout your microdosing protocol—regardless of whether they knew you were doing it—so they can gauge any changes.

## Exploring the Spectrum of Psychedelic Experiences

Another way to gauge your experience with microdosing is to use the time between microdosing protocols to see what else psychedelics have to offer. While microdosing, you may come to view psychedelics in purely practical, everyday terms. And while this perspective has many benefits—not least that it facilitates acceptance of microdosing by the relative mainstream—it only gives part of the picture. After all, long before the current explosion of interest in microdosing, psychedelics transformed lives profoundly through discrete, usually one-time mystical experiences.

So, how do you balance microdosing and macrodosing? How do you weave one into daily life as a biochemical aid and utilize the other to inspire psychospiritual inquiry? High doses encourage a more rigorous and comprehensive look at what everyday life means in the first place. Whereas microdosing is sub-perceptual, macrodosing is hyper-perceptual. Whereas one is practical and grounded in worldly activities, the other is philosophical, centered on questioning one's assumptions.

The two experiences aren't mutually exclusive, though; there's an interplay between them, by which insights from one can feed into the other. For example, full doses have the potential to meaningfully inform and direct a microdosing practice, complementing largely results-driven protocols with a deep reflective inquiry into the thought of who you wish to become.

For instance, on a full dose of psilocybin or LSD, you might realize the extent of dysfunction you've allowed to creep into certain relationships. After a full dose experience, you may feel empowered to address that dysfunction in your next cycle of microdosing. Conversely, while microdosing, you might discover things about yourself, such as ingrained resistances, deep-seated alienation, historical trauma, and so forth, that you'd like to explore in more detail. In this case, you can set a clear intention to do so before going on a macrodose experience.

At a more practical level, gaining experience with macrodoses can help you negotiate the full range of experiences you may have while microdosing. Let's say your microdose turns out to deliver a higher dose than you anticipated, you will know how to ride out the experience. In addition, knowing what to expect can prevent you from reacting with shock, confusion, and even panic, if an accidental trip is undesirable.

Of course, macrodoses have lasting benefits, quite apart from microdosing. In addition to the sometimes life-changing insights and realizations gleaned from the trip itself, people commonly report an "afterglow" effect—a noticeably brighter mood and higher levels of compassion, empathy, and self-esteem—that lasts for days, weeks, or even months afterward. Experiencing these positive emotional states can be especially useful for people who suffer from depression and social anxiety.

## Preparing for Your Macrodose

Before taking a high dose, remember that it requires more careful and thorough preparation than microdosing. If you wish to avoid a negative experience, optimize your mindset and surroundings beforehand—your "set and setting."

They include:

- Allowing at least one day on either side of your trip to prepare for and integrate the experience, ideally in nature.[110]
- Ensuring your space is clean and uncluttered or, if outside, as calm and pleasant as possible.

- Choosing music to facilitate your desired state of mind, avoiding harsh, jarring sounds and pessimistic lyrics.
- Finding a responsible sitter, at least for your first time—someone with the time, patience, and personal experience to reassure you if things go wrong.

Above all, do your research. Like microdosing, macrodosing isn't for everyone. However, if you've had success with microdosing and want to forge a stronger relationship with psychedelics, then taking a macrodose can be a transformative and rewarding next step—potentially also laying the foundations for your next cycle of microdosing.

## Macrodosing Integration Protocol

Microdosing and macrodosing can be part of your psychedelic use, much like regular brushing and home dental care fill in the gaps between visits to the dentist. Macrodosing addresses the deep-seated neuroses and problems, while microdosing, best when coupled with other mindfulness practices like breathwork and yoga, keeps everything running smoothly. In the wake of high-dose experiences, microdosing keeps that window of neuroplasticity open for a bit longer, helping the user weave in new behavioral patterns.

After higher dose sessions, there's often so much insight, energy, chaos, and sometimes even sorrow that it can be challenging to land afterward. Microdosing can help keep that swirling energy from getting stuck. Suppose you're interested in using microdosing as an integration tool after a high-dose experience. In that case, I suggest waiting at least one week after the high dose before microdosing, especially if you are new to psychedelics. We don't have the data yet to recommend a definitive duration for this time off or whether it's necessary. We know that a regular dose of LSD clears the system within a day, although specific metabolites can last longer. Microdosing may lead to a tolerance buildup over time, which is why it's helpful to create space between experiences.

After a week of integration post-high-dose journey, commit to microdosing two times per week for a minimum of thirty days. Always listen to your body and intuition when it's time to take a few weeks off to have some space and tune in.

When using multiple substances within a high-dose/microdosing regimen, the default is to stick to one substance. So, if you do a journey dose of psilocybin mushrooms, then microdose mushrooms as an integration tool. The same goes for LSD, San Pedro, and even ayahuasca. As you gain more experience and expertise, you will feel safe in relying even more on your discernment and intuition.


## When to Microdose Again?

One important question remains in this chapter: when should you restart your microdosing protocol?

After my initial seven months, I stopped doing any intentional microdosing protocol for approximately one year. During that period, I microdosed from time to time—usually with friends in the woods or at an awe-inspiring museum—but did not follow a regimen.

I chose to begin another microdosing protocol while planning for an extensive public speaking tour. Based on my original experience with microdosing, I knew my ability to articulate concepts and ideas improved while on small amounts of LSD.

It often takes some time to transform our relationship to these recurring patterns. For example, during my first seven months of microdosing with LSD, I was beginning to explore several ideas: What does it mean to perform? What does it mean to be productive? What does it mean to have ambition, and not just in the tangible way of building a business, but in a philosophical way? How do I listen when my soul is crying out for something different? And can microdosing help with those things?

For three or four years, the core North Star of my microdosing intention was based in business growth and social anxiety reduction. I wanted to become more comfortable with vulnerability and allow my entire self to be seen. I'm still leaning into these edges today.

When my business grew, I started getting into public speaking and felt blocked by my social anxiety. There's so much room for failure and shame when public speaking. I found that microdosing LSD before giving talks helped me to regulate my fear and stay more centered and present while on stage. Because microdosing activates the prefrontal cortex, I was more articulate in my delivery of concepts and ideas and found it easy to be flexible: I could drop into a practical, step-by-step, linear way of communicating, and I could just as quickly shift into storytelling mode, presenting moving experiences. So now, most days, when I speak in public, I take a microdose. It helps me drop into my center and hold space for the many hundred people in front of me.

Back to the core question: when to start again? Your intention is the most critical aspect when determining whether it's time to start another microdosing protocol. Do you have a specific reason to try microdosing again? Have you set a boundary of time and clear benchmarks to measure whether microdosing has been effective? Do you have a clear plan to integrate other beneficial habits with your follow-up microdosing protocols to not become psychologically reliant on it?

When refining your protocol, you may also choose to expand your repertoire of medicines. For example, once you've gotten familiar with LSD and psilocybin, you may want to branch out into ayahuasca or San Pedro (always doing so under proper care and guidance). Expanding variability with medicine work brings about a sense of novelty and a new appreciation for the practice.

Above all, think of microdosing as another tool that helps to amplify certain states of being that are elicited through practices like breathwork or meditation. Refining your precise protocol becomes intuitive when you focus less on the particulars, and more on the effect you wish to create.

## Want to Go Deeper?

Check out your Microdosing Mastery portal for exclusive resources, articles, and interviews to discover more about the topics from this chapter.

Just go to thethirdwave.co/bonus to access your exclusive book bonuses.

# PART III

# What Microdosing Makes Possible

# 10

# Clinical and Therapeutic Applications

After appearing on *The Tim Ferriss Show* in March 2015, Dr. Fadiman's following exploded. Fadiman and his co-researcher, Sophia Korb, leveraged this surge in public awareness to conduct an essential piece of observational research that would pave the way for future researchers to investigate the effects of microdosing.

In 2017, Fadiman and Korb sent a survey to their rapidly growing network, asking people to document their microdosing experiences at home. The survey asked participants to report the effects of microdosing on their mood and energy and their use of psychedelics for anxiety, depression, addiction, and post-traumatic stress disorder. They collected scores from 418 volunteers who had microdosed with psilocybin or LSD.[111]

Fadiman and Korb presented their findings at a 2017 MAPS Psychedelic Science conference in Oakland, California; Fadiman described the survey as more "search" than "research." The survey didn't dive into one specific indication but instead asked a wide range of questions about how people used psychedelics and the effects they experienced. As Fadiman told the crowd of over five hundred researchers and clinicians, this survey intended to create an umbrella for clinical researchers to find new questions to study microdosing.

Fadiman and Korb found that microdosing had a statistically significant effect on depression while improving energy and mood; on the other hand, it heightened anxiety at times. Though microdosing contraindicates lithium, the study found that people could microdose psilocybin or LSD in conjunction with almost every supplement or psychiatric medication.

This survey was the first step in a greater exploration of the landscape of microdosing and how it could impact people. Since then, studies have investigated the efficacy of microdosing for alleviating depression, replacing SSRIs, and treating PTSD, ADHD, and addiction. This chapter will look at a few pioneering studies that establish microdosing's potential clinical and therapeutic applications and those studies' limitations. We're still exploring the promise of these tools, but the future looks bright.

## Expanding the Reach of Research

Taking a cue from Fadiman and Korb, another group of researchers spearheaded by Rotem Petranker and Thomas M. Anderson conducted a more extensive survey out of the University of Toronto in 2019.[112] This study surveyed participants on the microdosing subreddit, which had grown from fifteen thousand users to more than one hundred thousand users due to widespread media coverage of microdosing. This survey expanded upon Fadiman and Korb's, including asking what concerns users grappled with—legality being the overwhelming majority.

The results were similar to those in Fadiman and Korb's study, showing significant improvements in mood and energy, alleviation of depressive symptoms, and a possible elevation in anxiety. These outcomes further developed microdosing's credibility, as it helped to better pinpoint microdosing's effects on people.

The next noteworthy study came through the Microdose.me app by Quantified Citizens, which allows users to track and log information regarding their doses and experiences and report the measures of specific variables and outcomes.[113]

Again, the results showed that microdosing alleviated depression symptoms by elevating mood and energy. *Nature*, one of the most prestigious scientific journals globally, published the findings. What makes this research noteworthy is its sample size of four thousand people, which is large compared to the other studies. The expanded pool of volunteers was primarily thanks to an interview Paul Stamets gave about the survey on *The Joe Rogan Experience* podcast.

The other noteworthy part of this study is that it used smartphones to track how microdosing interacts with a person's day-to-day life. By recording their observations on a device in their own pockets, volunteers could pinpoint certain variables in their real-time microdose usages, such as dose frequency, dose size, and support—or lack thereof.

This survey allowed researchers to uncover realistic behaviors and effects, away from the limitations of a more strict, rigorous clinical framework—an appropriate method to look at microdosing practices intended to be intuitive and custom-tailored for each person's needs.

## Working with Anxiety

Throughout these studies, LSD proved helpful for treating ADHD and depression, whereas psilocybin helped alleviate depression, anxiety, and addiction. However, both substances can increase anxiety, though that outcome can be reduced with careful attention to set and setting or through engaging with a professional microdosing coach. A coach can help navigate any anxiety that comes up in the process or help discern if the anxiety is rooted in something that needs to be confronted rather than managed. Sometimes the solution is as simple as needing to adjust a dose for an individual's needs.

At times, anxiety can bloom into fear or paranoia. Many people who struggle with rigidity in their lives are interested in psychedelics to loosen up. Still, this can be a double-edged sword, as psychedelics can also heighten paranoia. In that case, small doses, ideally with the aid of a professional, can help someone deal with the root cause of their rigidity and ultimately find peace.

## Weaning Off Psychiatric Medications

One of the most promising uses for microdosing psychedelics is to weave them into a medical context. This can assist people who want to get off their psychiatric medications when appropriate.

One such noteworthy case study on this topic conducted by Third Wave follows "Susan," a woman in her sixties who used psilocybin to stave off bouts of depression.[114] She had been using antidepressants for over six years. While they effectively treated her depression, they also numbed her other emotions. She wanted to find a way to manage her debilitating bouts of depression, which would arise about every three months, and still experience the range of human emotion. So, she discontinued Prozac, and within six months, her depression was back, along with anxiety.

Susan started microdosing psilocybin to counteract these bouts of depression. She found that she required a slightly higher microdosing amount due to her previous SSRI use and her age. So, she took 0.5 grams of dried mushrooms every three days, an average "museum dose" rather than a classic microdose. The psilocybin was a prophylactic that protected her against the events that normally triggered a depressive crash.

While it comes down to the individual—and there are exceptions to any rule—it is common for older people to need a higher dose. Sometimes this is due to previous medication use, like in Susan's case. But often, the rigidity built over decades impacts sensitivity to the medicine. Hence, a higher dose is initially necessary for the person to feel the psilocybin. Then, after its effects are recognizable and the person opens to the medicine, it's easier to adjust the dose.

Susan's approach of essentially replacing her SSRI was an unconventional way to microdose. Usually, microdosing is an integrative tool, not something meant to be taken consistently. Rather, it is more typically taken for a month at a time, followed by a break. But the main point for everyone is to heal, and by microdosing in this way, Susan was able to keep her depression in check without numbing her other experiences.

Consuming lower doses of psilocybin on a somewhat regular basis can help rewire the brain by spurring new dendritic growth and improving energy and mood. It's advisable for those looking to use microdosing to wean off or replace pharmaceuticals to do so with a trained coach or clinician. In the same way, therapists and coaches can help facilitate a high-dose experience. Their support can help guide you to your desired outcome in a microdosing protocol.

## Working with Addiction

Sometimes good mental health comes down to deconditioning and letting go of negative thought patterns and behaviors. Addiction is an obvious example, and some have been able to manage it through microdosing. One Reddit user, for instance, found they were suddenly able to "mindfully and joyfully accomplish tasks" they'd otherwise have drunk alcohol for.[115] Others have found their cravings substantially diminished.

In 2014, Johns Hopkins published an open-label study in which psychedelics showed an 80 percent efficacy for helping participants quit smoking, making psilocybin more than twice as effective as the current leading medications to treat nicotine addiction.[116] These results were so promising that the National Institutes of Health gave its first grant to psychedelic therapy, specifically to explore the efficacy of psilocybin for nicotine addiction treatment.

One of the reasons psychedelics are so effective at healing addiction is their biological and psychospiritual impact. Biologically, psychedelics interrupt rigidity by creating new plasticity and dendritic growth, which improves attention, mood, and energy. Psychospiritually, especially at higher doses, psychedelics can usher in a "come to Jesus" moment where a person must confront something they've been denying or repressing, such as the extent and harm of their nicotine addiction. Because psychedelic experiences often make people face the notion of death, it's common for users to come out of the experience more inspired to thrive in their daily lives. Psychedelic experiences can serve as the impetus they need to quit smoking.

Nicotine and caffeine are two of the most widely used drugs globally. They've been legal for many years and were central to the Industrial Revolution because of their impact on focus and the convergent thinking that was so important for hundreds of years. Now, our world is largely different, and we're seeing stimulants add to the problem of anxiety rather than simply increasing productivity. Currently, the overabundance and overuse of stimulants negatively impact our quality of life.

One member of the Third Wave community, "Jane," was a mid-career project manager and tended to self-medicate by smoking cigarettes.[117] She kept trying to quit but was repeatedly drawn back by everyday stress. Cigarette and coffee breaks offered her a reprieve from stressful situations at work or dealing with family.

Jane had some significant experiences with psychedelics, particularly San Pedro and ayahuasca. She was confused because the benefits she experienced through those high-dose experiences helped her grow emotionally and spiritually. However, she still couldn't quit smoking even though she knew she needed to. Her dependence on cigarettes and all its accompanying rituals was too strong.

She enrolled in a Third Wave microdosing course and intended to reduce her caffeine and nicotine intake. Creating her intention and choosing her setting made a massive difference in her journey.

She followed up her intention by taking 0.1 to 0.15 grams of psilocybin every third day, which helped calm her mood and reduced her urge to reach for a cigarette.

The positive effects of microdosing extended into her off days as well. On the off days immediately following a microdose, she noticed an increased activation of her senses. She was more alert, brighter, and more energized on the second day than on the first, which interrupted the cycle of substance dependence. In addition, she automatically found her cravings more manageable.

The results were even more evident upon visiting her family, a situation that usually triggered cigarette cravings. By following Third Wave's microdosing protocols, she managed the stress and stayed present in the situation. She said, "The whole atmosphere while there was a lot more gentle. There was a calmness that I'd never experienced before."

Jane layered microdoses onto a preexisting mindfulness practice. She believed the synergy of the two would transform her, that the combination of medicine and mindfulness would positively affect her neural pathways. The most significant change was being more present in her conscious awareness. She reported she no longer ruminates about the past or worries about the future. After this experience, Jane could navigate stressful or triggering situations without resorting to nicotine or caffeine.

This case study highlights the synergistic effects of psilocybin consumption and mindfulness. In neurobiology, psychedelics and medication decreased activity in the brain's default mode network, responsible for self-referential processes, otherwise known as the ego or sense of self. When we disrupt our sense of self, we can better observe the present moment from a nonjudgmental point of view, creating more space for psychological flexibility.

## Understanding Placebo in Psychedelics

A study out of the Imperial College in London showed no statistical significance in results between participants who microdosed psychedelics and those who took a placebo. These results seem to contradict the thousands of respondents of previous microdosing surveys. But rather than a lack of efficacy in psychedelic use, I would argue this study highlights a fatal flaw in research designs for studying microdosing.

The Imperial College study was self-blinded. Therefore, the subjects didn't know whether they were taking a real microdose or a placebo, and they self-reported results. As I mentioned, the results showed no statistical significance between the actual doses and the placebos. But, in reviewing the study's methodology, the researchers did little to account for each individual's dosage requirements, and it was hard for subjects to control their dosages. Furthermore, there was no emphasis on supporting practices to cultivate intention or to seek guidance from professionals.

As previously discussed, microdosing is a nonspecific amplifier. When given nothing to amplify through support or intention, the practice will inevitably show less efficacy than if done with proper backing. Therefore, any research exploring the placebo effect of microdosing must require accountability and support from trained professionals. Intention and reflection are central to the success of a microdosing protocol. In this way, this study fell dramatically short.

On the flip side of placebo assumptions, many studies have proven an active response from the body when consuming micro-doses of LSD, starting at six micrograms. Other studies show that a dose of twenty micrograms effectively treats conditions such as ADHD and depression. However, for analyses to be accurate, we need to refine protocols, enhance how people are using them, and improve overall training and methodology specific to how micro-dosing can be combined with various nonpsychedelic modalities.

To explore the efficacy of psychedelics compared to placebo in the proper context, it's helpful to explore how the efficacy of SSRIs has waned over time.

When SSRIs first came out in the 1980s, they showed signif-icant clinical efficacy. But as the population grew accustomed to working with SSRIs, the effectiveness dropped. Recent findings in 2019–2020 showed that SSRIs and placebo are equally effective, helping about 40 percent of users. Essentially, SSRIs are now no more effective than placebo.

This decline could be explained by a population that has been constantly and sometimes over-prescribed these medications. Another contributor to the waning efficacy is the powerful placebo effect held by advertising the "great new thing" that will solve everyone's problems. For better or worse, SSRIs are no longer the "great new thing."

We realize now that the underlying science was flawed in developing many of these conventional psychiatric treatments. Researchers sought to treat the brain like they would treat an infection; they sought a neurological equivalent of penicillin. But of course, the brain doesn't work the same way as the gut. Now, more than three decades later, we understand so much more about neurology. We now know that neuroplasticity is key to human adaptation. The need for a more effective method to treat clinical conditions is fostering the current psychedelic renaissance.

At present, the approach to microdosing research is not as fleshed out and mature as high-dose clinical research. A proper research study must include professional guides to manage consumption and protocols even with lower doses. If researchers applied that same level of integrity to micro-dosing research, we'd see more statistically significant outcomes, just as we're seeing with high-dose, psychotherapy-assisted research.

As personalized medicine grows, we'll understand more about individualized dosages. We've seen that some people need just 0.1 gram of mushrooms to see a positive change in their daily lives, while others need much more. We have yet to study how people intuitively and scientifically adapt their protocol with proper support. It will be impossible to measure the impact of low-dose psychedelics accurately until then. People are actively working toward this now, but we're still in the early days of available technology. It will be three to five years before the technology can scientifically validate appropriate microdosing protocols for greater efficacy.

## The Rise of the Decentralized Nutraceutical Industry

Currently, there are two core types of companies flourishing in the microdosing sphere. One is biotech companies that create synthetic forms of psilocybin and LSD to treat various conditions, including inflammation, depression, addiction, and ADHD. Tens of millions of dollars have gone into microdosing research to understand whether psychedelics could replace traditional psychiatric medications within the next seven to ten years. These psychedelics would be prescribed through a medical model and covered by insurance, just like the framework for our current medicines.

The second type of company is nutraceutical companies focused on formulations with herbs and mushrooms in supplement form. These are mainly in Canada, though there are others throughout the United States. They create formulations with psilocybin stacked with other herbs and mushrooms such as lion's mane, cordyceps, ashwagandha, rhodiola, reishi, and so on. These supplements aim to help with performance, sensuality, mood enhancement, and more, which creates an implicit intention when someone ingests the supplement.

These formulations help us reclaim the herbalist inside of us and use natural medicines, which are powerful and effective in supporting the nervous system. This promotes emotional well-being, neurogenesis, and neuroplasticity. This approach will grow in scope and accessibility over the next few years as governments decriminalize psychedelics, especially in the United States.

Accessibility and safe availability of microdosing through a clinical model are essential. Psilocybin truffles have been available in the Netherlands for years with no public health consequences. But many people believe that going from illegal to widely accessible under a dispensary model in the US could lead to chaos. Making microdosing supplements available through a clinical model mitigates that risk and allows people to develop an intuitive relationship with these substances.

Building an intuitive, safe relationship with psychedelics is important. Microdosing in a clinical environment with trained professionals can bring many participants a sense of significant ease, to say nothing of the results gleaned from these experiences and shared with the population at large. As people explore the power of psychedelics, they may very well find microdosing helps mitigate risks associated with higher doses because of the established relationship between the user and the substance. In addition, widely accessible, high-quality formulations will help people feel alive, vibrant, and energized when we increasingly need to access our life force and energy.

## Microdosing and Psychotherapy

At present, most studies on psychedelics and psychotherapy focus on guided high-dose experiences. Yet, anecdotally we know that microdosing has also worked within a psychotherapeutic context. "My microdosing has been in conjunction with therapy to address my depression/anxiety issues, so my positive results have been a two-pronged attack on these issues," a Third Wave reader wrote. "I have had therapy by itself in the past and the results I have found this time have been much more groundbreaking for me and in a much more timely manner. There are a lot of variables with these results but I truly believe that microdosing has been an integral part of the positive outcome for these issues."

The sheer extent of evidence showing that LSD and psilocybin can be helpful for mental disorders helps explain why many people find microdosing productive.

The existing research on psychedelics is compelling, especially given the difficulty of conducting studies with Schedule I substances strictly controlled under federal law. Microdosing is hard to examine because any practical research would require the subjects to possess the substances and self-administer—which is currently illegal. A potential loosening of legal restrictions could mean a vast wave of new research, providing a deeper understanding of what these chemicals can do and how they act on the human brain.

In turn, this research may reveal how microdosing can offer positive holistic health effects and even, as some people have reported, save lives.

## Want to Go Deeper?

Check out your Microdosing Mastery portal for exclusive resources, articles, and interviews to discover more about the topics from this chapter.

Just go to thethirdwave.co/bonus to access your exclusive book bonuses.

# 11

# Enhancing Creativity and Flow

As helpful and therapeutic as microdosing may be, many leaders find the practice appealing. This focus is not for what it can fix but for what it can make possible: a more creative and fulfilling life, personally and professionally.

As an entrepreneur searching for a better way to approach work, mitigate procrastination, and boost productivity, I began microdosing in July 2015, around the same time other entrepreneurs began tuning in.

Before 2015, only a handful of folks knew about microdosing. This widespread growth in recognition came because of Dr. Jim Fadiman's appearance on the Tim Ferriss podcast. In turn, this led to experimental microdosing among some of the most powerful and innovative tech entrepreneurs in Silicon Valley.

## Microdosing for Creativity

In an interview with CNN Money, author and venture capitalist Tim Ferriss suggested there was a specific reason that Silicon Valley culture was at the forefront of the microdosing movement. "The billionaires I know, almost without exception, use hallucinogens on a regular basis," Ferriss said. "[They're] trying to be very disruptive and look at the problems in the world…and ask completely new questions."[118]

In his posthumous biography, Apple co-founder Steve Jobs famously claimed that taking LSD was such a profound experience that it ranked as one of the most important things he ever did. Considering his business success, that's a powerful statement. It may be tempting to dismiss Jobs as an outlier, a visionary fated for significant accomplishments no matter his formative experiences. However, it's more difficult to ignore the sheer volume of reports on how completely psychedelics in general—and now microdosing, specifically—have permeated the culture and workforce in Silicon Valley. They have undoubtedly played a role in developing many apps and products that people around the world use every day.

It can be challenging to get a handle on just how widespread the practice is because psychedelics are still illegal under federal and state laws in the US. Understandably, many people are reluctant to speak publicly about their use, though word is getting out. In earlier chapters, we outlined transparent accounts in mainstream publications like *Rolling Stone*, *Wired*, *Forbes*, *BBC*, the *New York Times*, the *Washington Post*, the *Guardian,* and *GQ,* which suggests that reluctance to speak out is fading.

The prevalence of psychedelic use among some of the most prominent and successful people in Silicon Valley has the potential to make a dramatic impact on reducing or eliminating psychedelic stigma. As more and more people acknowledge having tried microdosing and found it helpful, psychedelics may be able to shed the bad juju they acquired through decades of negative propaganda proffered by the media and the US government.

Some people have already been willing to go on the record about their microdosing. For example, longtime Cisco engineer Kevin Herbert acknowledged to CNN that using LSD helped him solve complicated work problems, and many of his younger colleagues also use psychedelics to improve their output and creativity.[119] The practice is also growing in other high-profile fields, as athletes, actors, and writers credit microdosing with helping them break out of ruts and achieve new levels of performance.

More privately, many individuals have shared the profound benefits of microdosing with Third Wave. These anecdotal reports parallel executives and celebrities who practice microdosing to help meet their personal and professional goals. For example, one reader described intense focus during writing sessions while microdosing:

I am very focused for 2–4 hours, depending on how tired I am leading up to the dose. During the dose, I'm very, very slightly loopy—my thoughts are mostly coherent and streamlined, but I usually wait until

I'm sober again to double-check my work. One noticeable difference is that, when I write to the point that I need to fact-check or research something, I will do that and then return to writing. Ordinarily, this can either halt my flow, or I will add a marker and come back to it.

Another contributor noted, "I can focus more easily on complex tasks such as writing an essay as I can almost 'feel' how my thoughts move through my hand on to my pen and then on to the paper."

The more people speak about microdosing and using psychedelics, the more firmly the concept will seep into mainstream thought. This is because we are coming to see microdosing not as something subversive or dangerous but as a valuable tool to help unlock human effectiveness.

## Psychedelics and Tech Innovation

As indicated prior, Silicon Valley is a natural location for the epicenter of microdosing. Before federal prohibition, the Bay Area was a hotbed of legal LSD experimentation. Many of the people who became giants in the tech field used LSD in their formative years and developed breakthrough computer technologies. "From the start, a small but significant crossover existed between those who were experimenting with drugs and the burgeoning tech community in San Francisco," reports *The Economist's 1843 Magazine.*[120] Today's microdosing community continues the relationship between psychedelics and high tech that started decades ago.

That relationship has contributed to some game-changing innovations, including the personal computer and the computer mouse. And no wonder—the idealism of pioneers who envisioned computers as a tool to empower the individual with egalitarian access to information is reminiscent of aspirations frequently attached to psychedelic consumption—to free human minds from their constraints. Arguably, LSD played a vital role in developing the personal computer, which went on to irrevocably alter the very nature of work and human interactions in the ensuing decades.[121]

And the ubiquitous computer mouse? In the book *What the Dormouse Said*, journalist John Markoff relates the comparative history between psychedelics and software engineers and how the Bay Area counterculture of the '60s and '70s, steeped with LSD, bled over into the nascent tech scene.[122] For example, Doug Engelbart, inventor of the mouse, was a veteran of the International Foundation for Advanced Study's LSD experiments and founded the Augmented Human Intellect Research Center at the Stanford Research Institute.

Today we can see the spreading popularity of psychedelics in gatherings like Burning Man, which attracts entrepreneurs in droves. As groundbreaking entrepreneur Elon Musk said in an interview with Re/code, "If you haven't been, you just don't get Silicon Valley."[123] For many who attend the extended art festival held annually in the Nevada desert, psychedelics are essential to expressing their creativity and culture in a nonjudgmental environment.

But is there a connection between dreaming up better ways of solving computer problems and performing art in the desert? There seems to be. "I like going to Burning Man," Google CEO Larry Page said at the Google I/O conference. "An environment where people can try new things. I think as technologists we should have some safe places where we can try out new things and figure out the effect on society. What's the effect on people, without having to deploy it to the whole world."[124]

## From Silicon Valley to the Collective Consciousness

Entrepreneurs may be among the most vocal supporters of using psychedelics to enhance performance, but the benefits have been experienced far beyond the Santa Clara Valley. For instance, lore from extreme sports culture in the '60s and '70s is rife with stories of people using LSD to get the most from their bodies and minds. Psychedelics were a natural fit with extreme sports competitors, many of whom were veterans of the hippie movement of the '60s. They often saw themselves as rebels or outlaws.

"LSD can increase your reflex time to lightning speed, improve your balance to the point of perfection, increase your concentration …and make you impervious to weakness or pain," writer James Oroc claimed in a report for the Multidisciplinary Association for Psychedelic Studies.[125] "Various experienced individuals have climbed some of the hardest big walls in Yosemite, heli-skied first descents off Alaskan peaks, competed in world-class snowboarding competitions, raced motocross bikes, surfed enormous Hawaiian waves, flown hang-gliders above 18,000 feet, or climbed remote peaks in the Rockies, the Alps, the Andes, and even above 8,000 meters in the Himalayas—all while under the influence of LSD."

In a more conventional setting, Pittsburgh Pirates pitcher Dock Ellis famously claimed that he was on LSD when he threw a no-hitter in 1970. And outside of sports, countless bands and musicians, including The Beatles, The Rolling Stones, Grateful Dead, Jefferson Airplane, and many more cited LSD and other psychedelics for helping spark their creativity to write and perform music.

As general awareness of psychedelics expands, microdosing provides a palatable way for people concerned about psychoactive reactions and hallucinations to consider the other benefits of LSD, mescaline, psilocybin, and ayahuasca. Framing their use as a tool to access flow states provides another way to combat the stigma attached to psychedelics in the United States. The tipping point must be close; after all, very few people in America or other developed countries could say they haven't consumed media, used a piece of software, or watched an athletic performance that psychedelics have influenced.

And now, the reach of these substances is spreading even further, largely thanks to information shared on popular podcasts. Tim Ferriss, an active proponent of psychedelics and their benefits, hosted one podcast on how psychedelics could be at the forefront of the next big medical breakthrough, then followed it with another show that looked specifically at microdosing.[126] He interviewed microdosing trailblazer Dr. Fadiman on that episode. "[People who microdose] can be creative longer," Fadiman told Ferriss. "Kind of steady, more in flow."[127]

Joe Rogan, a comedian and popular podcast host, has dedicated several episodes to exploring the experiences and breakthroughs his guests have experienced using psychedelics. In one episode, he talks specifically about microdosing with author and ethnopharmacologist Dennis McKenna, brother of renowned psychedelic explorer Terence McKenna.[128] "People are using psilocybin these days in what they call microdosing, taking very small doses and seeing these profound benefits," Rogan says.

He speaks of his friend who takes doses before kickboxing and claims he can see things before they happen in the ring. "It's almost like he's reading people's minds before they're about to do something," says Rogan.

McKenna replies that he's not surprised at all. "[Psilocybin] is a lens through which you can look at the world and see aspects of it that are always there, but you've never noticed it before, because we're programmed not to," he explains. "They can reverse this background foreground relationship that we're so used to. Suddenly what's right in front of you is not so important and you can pay attention to the things in the background that you're programmed to suppress and ignore."

"They teach different ways of perception," McKenna continues.

"You realize there's a different way to be in the world. There's a different way to perceive what you experience that normally you don't."

Before now, who would have put kickboxing and microdosing together? Yet, microdosing is spreading into every corner of the globe, with potentially profound implications for the trajectory of humanity.

## Psychedelics Help to Tap True Potential

Some experts argue that increased psychedelic use will lead human beings to conquer completely new horizons.

The book *Stealing Fire: How Silicon Valley, the Navy SEALs, and Maverick Scientists Are Revolutionizing the Way We Live and Work* by Steven Kotler and Jamie Wheal explores the history of psychedelics and how they help people tap into their true potential. Within its pages, the authors muse about what might come next.[129]

"As far back as we can trace Western civilization, buried among the stories that bore schoolchildren to tears, we find tales of rebel upstarts willing to bet it all for an altered state of consciousness," the authors write.

Today, as more people explore ways of altering their consciousness, the possibilities of what we can create have expanded to a surprising degree. "We are witnessing a groundswell, a growing movement to storm heaven and steal fire," the book states. "It's a revolution in human possibility."

By altering our connection with the ego through psychedelics, meditation, trances, virtual reality, or other means, we free the body and spirit to develop new ideas outside the default framework of human thought. "With our self forever standing guard over our ideas, crazy schemes and hare-brained notions tend to get filtered out long before they can become useful," *Stealing Fire* explains. "But intoxication lessens those constraints."

"When we consistently see more of 'what is really happening,' we can liberate ourselves from the limitations of our psychology," the authors describe. "We can put our egos to better use, using them to modulate our neurobiology and with it, our experience. We can train our brains to find our minds."

Silicon Valley, of course, is a prime testing ground for crazy schemes and hare-brained notions. Combining the limitless potential of technology with human beings pushing themselves beyond their ordinary peripheries through microdosing and other techniques opens the door to boundless possibilities for our future.

## Microdosing for Flow States

Proponents of microdosing say that taking regular, sub-perceptible psychedelic doses enhances their performance, whether their task is to improve code or develop creative business solutions. The practice works by inducing *flow states* in users, a phrase coined by psychologist Mihaly Csikszentmihalyi to investigate optimal human experience.[130] In other words, the substances help people focus on creative endeavors, with a dramatic effect on the ability to remain mindful.

This phenomenon speaks to the importance of dose calibration. We all know that LSD is a complete inebriant that creates chaotic, intense situations at high doses. No one would ever want to be in a position that challenges their physical safety while taking a high dose of LSD. But when that dose level is calibrated to a specific intention for alertness and coordination, improved movement, and general awareness, a microdose becomes a beautiful tool to help reach a flow state.

Just as a high dose of psychedelics doesn't guarantee a life-changing mystical experience, a microdose doesn't guarantee entry into a flow state. Still, it's one of the best methodologies for a repeatable, replicable experience.

Though flow states can be elusive, people notice that micro-dosing makes flow more accessible by helping the user break free of rigidity. In other words, microdosing is an exogenous means of opening the doorway to get into the zone. The description of "being in the zone" that many extreme sports participants attribute to LSD and other psychedelics echoes the flow state described by Silicon Valley microdosing enthusiasts.

In practice, flow means improved concentration and creativity, resulting in developing novel ideas to solve complex problems—a perfect tool for a software entrepreneur or anyone in a professional field that requires innovation or insight.

For example, a freelancer wrote to Third Wave to describe the benefits of getting into a flow state: "While I was working on a project during the day I'm microdosing, I used to give it much more effort and time and I was really enjoying what I'm doing without getting lost somewhere else or taking breaks from time to time, I was living at the moment without any distraction from outside. Yeah, it made what I do more enjoyable."

As I've mentioned before, the most authoritative source of information about microdosing yet compiled is Dr. James Fadiman's book, *The Psychedelic Explorer's Guide*.[131] Fadiman provides a suggested protocol for microdosing and has been collecting reports for several years about how psychedelics have affected his readers. "In low doses, they facilitate awareness of solutions to technical and artistic problems," he notes.

People who followed his protocol wrote to him about how microdosing improved their concentration:

"Was able to shut out virtually all distracting influences," one report said.

"I was impressed with the intensity of concentration, the forcefulness and exuberance with which I could proceed toward the solution," another wrote.

A third user had a similar experience. "My experience during the session was an unbelievable increase in the ability to concentrate and make decisions. It was impossible to procrastinate. Cobwebs, blocks, and binds disappeared."

Fadiman's respondents reported increases in their creativity as well. "I've found that I've had some brilliant outbursts (at least they seemed brilliant to me) with respect to both work product and personal creative projects," one wrote in. "What seems to happen is that the 'flow' state described by Mihaly Csikszentmihalyi and frequently noted in the sports arena is a lot easier to access and stay in."

Other respondents said they found similar results. "Sub-doses of ten to twenty micrograms allow me to increase my focus, open my heart, and achieve breakthrough results while remaining integrated within my routine," one reader said.

"I would venture to say that my wit, response time, and visual and mental acuity seem greater than normal on it," another wrote.

Third Wave readers also reported overall positive results. For example, in one Third Wave survey, 25.5 percent of fifty-one respondents said they noticed improved problem-solving after microdosing. In a second survey, 229 individuals ranked microdosing's impact on various aspects of their performance on a scale of one to six. Respondents gave an average score of 4.65 for span of focus, 4.57 for problem-solving, and 4.76 for creativity. For general mood, microdosers reported an average score of 5.2.

One of the core requirements of flow is to engage with the right degree of challenge. To find the right difficulty level, follow the 4 percent rule, which means taking on tasks that are about 4 percent more challenging than usual. When using psychedelics to enhance your flow, keep in mind that each substance creates a slightly different effect. For example, if your challenging experience is somatic or emotional, psilocybin may be the better choice, as it can increase your sense of empathy and embodiment. If your goal is to increase performance or productivity, LSD may be the better choice. LSD is more dopaminergic than psilocybin, which means LSD increases focus, enhancing your ability to do deep research or tackle a complex project.

Once you choose the best substance for your intention, it's simply about dialing in a dose to find the sweet spot. You want to choose an amount where you can be open, playful, and creative while remaining grounded, focused, and stable. Staying centered is the key to entering flow.

## Related Benefits

Not everyone said that microdosing helped with focus or creativity, but many reported significant benefits. "I struggle with concentration and can be very irritable, microdosing greatly improves that for me," a real estate agent and US military veteran said in a survey sent out to Third Wave's microdosing community. Another report from a Dutch teacher stated, "At the end of the day, a wow feeling of everything that was accomplished."

An actor described how microdosing enhanced the ability to be present in the craft: "Conversation flowed beautifully, like my mind always found the words I was looking for. It was great for my acting ability too, and I felt much more present during challenging scenes."

Several people described the benefits of microdosing in collaborative work efforts: "My positivity has skyrocketed, and I feel that I put out such a positive energy force that I attracted positive results in my workplace—such as getting new clients, treating my staff better, the list can truly go on," said one individual.

"I was no longer sensitive to criticism or confrontations, my work ethic improved and I was much more open and caring for customers and coworkers. It became less about me and more about the collective," another reported.

"[It was] easier to work with, collaborate with colleagues," a reader wrote in, "even those who've been difficult in the past; better able to concentrate and connect all day rather than in fits and starts; clarity in presenting and a general overall sense of understanding and being able to communicate complex ideas."

## Results May Vary

While the sheer volume of anecdotal evidence is a testament to the results that microdosing offers to many people, not everyone who tries microdosing reports a positive experience or chooses to partake again. For example, reporters for *Vox* and the Seattle-based newspaper *The Stranger* tried microdosing themselves.

"At one point during my first session, I looked up and realized I'd been totally engrossed in my work with no real awareness of anything else for an hour," Baynard Woods wrote in *Vox* after taking a tiny hit of LSD. "I found myself more deeply absorbed in that zone we all hope to be in where the doer and the deed dissolve together into the pleasure of pure work."[132] However, he also reported a harrowing experience with night terrors after mixing microdosing with heavy alcohol use.

Though Katie Herzog in *The Stranger* didn't have the same experience as Woods, she came away from her experience feeling that microdosing LSD was not a solution for her anxiety. Though she felt it did benefit her work, she turned to therapy instead. Of her microdosing experience, she shared: "It's not uncommon for me to spend more time wandering than writing. But on that particular day, I didn't wander at all, and by the time I looked up, it was dark. This continued into the next day when I wasn't microdosing, and I still got more done in an afternoon than I had the previous week."[133]

Ultimately, both writers were ambivalent about their experiments. Nevertheless, their reports are an important reminder that microdosing isn't a magic potion that will automatically bring success and happiness to everyone. Instead, everyone must find their path to what works and feels comfortable.

## What We Know about Why It Works: Studies on How Microdosing Can Help Creativity, Focus, and Problem-Solving

As I've stated throughout this book, we do not have a vast body of scientific research that backs up the wave of anecdotal reports about the benefits of microdosing. However, certain studies of people taking high doses of psychedelics support the idea that these substances can improve creativity and problem-solving while providing hints as to the "why."

## Peak Problem-Solving

In 1966, Dr. Fadiman conducted research involving 200 mg of mescaline sulfate—equivalent to one hundred micrograms of LSD —given to twenty-seven subjects who worked mainly in science, math, and engineering.[134] He instructed each subject to focus on a tricky, unsolved professional problem. After ingesting the mescaline, participants spent three hours relaxing, followed by an hour of tests, and then they were given four hours to work on their problem.

The study staff gave participants several instructions to help them hone in on solutions. First, they told the subjects to try to identify the process at the center of the problem and then scan through any number of possible solutions, trusting the brain to intuit the correct answer. The staff reminded participants that they could see a bigger picture of the problem if they looked at the roadblock from a new perspective. That break from their ego, provided by the psychedelic, helped them seek the best answers based on merit while not worrying about saving face or salvaging previously failed approaches.

Nearly everyone who participated in the experiment reported enhanced problem-solving ability. In addition, over half of the participants conceptualized solutions to their problems, some with deep real-world applications. Among the results: breakthroughs in ideas or products such as space probe experiments, electron accelerators, a conceptual photon design, brick and mortar building designs, medical diagnoses, and a vibratory microtome (a tool to harvest very thin slices of animal and plant tissues or other materials).

In reports following the experiment, the subjects described eleven ways in which their experience enhanced their functioning. For some, the mescaline helped lower their inhibition or fear of failure. "Although doing well on these problems would be fine, failure to get ahead on them would be threatening. However, as it turned out, on this afternoon the normal blocks in the way of progress seemed to be absent," one of the participants said afterward.

Others said they could see their problems in a larger context, experiencing enhanced fluency and flexibility of ideation. "I could handle two or three different ideas at the same time and keep track of each," a subject claimed. "I also got the feeling that creativity is an active process in which you limit yourself and have an objective, so there is a focus about which ideas can cluster and relate," another said.

Participants' capacity for visual imagery and fantasy was enhanced, as was their ability to concentrate on their problems. "I was impressed with the intensity of concentration, the forcefulness and exuberance with which I could proceed toward the solution," one said.

Subjects also said they felt heightened empathy, allowing them to look at a situation from another person's eyes or in a new light. Such a perspective allowed them to grasp the problem and understand how objects and components function within it. They additionally reported an increased sense of empathy, further improving problem-solving capacity.

Participants noted that their brains' subconscious data was more accessible, and they could associate different ideas to help come to a breakthrough. Finally, they said they felt heightened motivation to obtain closure and could visualize the completed solution. "I visualized the result I wanted and subsequently brought the variables into play which could bring that result about," one said. "I had great visual (mental) perceptibility; I could imagine what was wanted, needed, or not possible with almost no effort. I was amazed at my idealism, my visual perception, and the rapidity with which I could operate."

"The practical value of obtained solutions is a check against subjective reports of accomplishment that might be attributable to temporary euphoria," the experiment concludes. "We are dealing with materials and experimental situations that have long-term effects; it would be foolhardy and irresponsible to treat this kind of research as if it were isolated from the fabric of the subjects' lives."

## Increased Insights and Innovations

Due to federal prohibition on psychedelics and the accompanying obstacles to scientific research, subsequent years have seen only a few follow-up experiments. However, anecdotal reports to support the research study's conclusion have surfaced from time to time.

In the book *LSD—The Problem-Solving Psychedelic*, P.G. Stafford and B.H. Golightly reveal the tale of a naval researcher who used LSD to develop a solution regarding the design of a submarine detection device.[135] After years of unsuccessfully working on the problem, he solved it ten minutes after taking the acid. His inspiration resulted in a patented device that the Navy used. In addition, the book describes advances in furniture design, visual arts, and writing experienced by people under the influence of LSD.

In another anecdotal take, researcher Dr. Jeremy Narby spoke with three molecular biologists after they took ayahuasca for the first time. Each responded that they had come to insights that would be useful for their professional research, largely around the fractal and unitive nature of reality, from cells to consciousness to the greater cosmos.

## Making New Associations

Researchers have recently compiled information that helps us understand how psychedelics encourage divergent thinking. For example, a 2016 study by the Beckley Foundation, "Ayahuasca and Creativity: the Amazonian Plant Brew Improves Divergent Thinking," provides evidence that the psychedelic drink made from Amazonian jungle plants can help people with their problem-solving abilities.[136] The research looks at how the substance impacts users' ability to think divergently—or outside the box—to consider possible solutions to a situation or problem.

The study assessed twenty-six participants by having them identify associations between cartoon pictures of animals and everyday objects. They tested the subjects before taking the ayahuasca and about two hours after drinking it. After ingesting the drink, participants developed more alternative associations between the pictures, demonstrating increased divergent thinking.

The researchers suggest that these substances are not responsible for creating these associations but for liberating the person's innate ability to make such connections. "It is important to bear in mind that psychedelics help us to make full use of our inborn creative capabilities, rather than…supplying us with additional creativity," the study's authors concluded.

This study is fascinating, and the researchers suggested further investigation to assess the subjects' mood under the hypothesis that a positive mindset would correlate to an uptick in divergent thinking. They also recommended evaluating the usefulness of the creative ideas generated under ayahuasca and tracking the longevity of the effects on divergent thinking.

In a similar vein, a University College London study suggested that LSD boosted the capacity for associative thinking. When asked to name objects they were shown, many subjects who took LSD erroneously misidentified the props by calling related things instead, for example, saying "foot" when shown an image of a shoe.[137]

"This study suggests that LSD puts our brains in a state similar to that found in dreaming, where thoughts become less logical and more associative," the *Psychedelic Scientist* article notes. "The increase in connectivity produced in the brain by LSD is amazingly complex, and results in profound changes in cognition."[138]

Third Wave readers also experienced the benefits of divergent thinking. "All topics become more interesting," a pharmacology student from Australia said. "Attention is increased as I subconsciously think of a problem from multiple angles."

"I felt like there was a click in my lens of perception. I thought about things from a different light, [a] different manner...all-around really enjoyable," reported another respondent to a Third Wave survey.

We don't know precisely how this "click" happens, but brain scans of people using LSD show that the chemical triggers activity all over the brain, allowing new pathways and connections to form. These brain scans could explain why psychedelics are so effective at lifting the restrictions of conventional thinking.[139]

The sum of the research on psychedelics as creative agents combined with thorough and convincing anecdotal reports suggests that humans require a catalyst or an instigator to function at highest capacity. By limiting the censors that govern conscious awareness, psychedelics can dramatically expand the possibilities of what human beings can accomplish. Microdosing is a promising way to advance toward divergent and associative thinking that could help scientists, entrepreneurs, and engineers solve complex problems.

## Other Ways to Access Flow States

Microdosing is the method that enabled me to overcome professional issues with procrastination and creative resistance. For the first time, I was able to execute consistently at the level of excellence that I wanted, leading to the growth and success of Third Wave.

I'm far from alone. In *Stealing Fire*, Steven Kotler and Jamie Wheal point out the prevalence of psychoactive substances across various species, from birds to baboons to dolphins to elephants. Drug-seeking behavior from the animal kingdom suggests a primary evolutionary drive toward altered, disruptive, or de-patterning states of consciousness. However, psychedelics are far from the only means for attaining them.

Kotler and Wheal say that achieving flow states requires selflessness (ego loss), timelessness (time dilation or contraction), effortlessness, and richness (vivid insights and detailed information).[140] They argue that by understanding their psychological and neurobiological basis, we can identify the best, most reliable means for their induction.

Sensory deprivation tanks, for example, in which people float on body-temperature saltwater in pitch-black darkness, also enhance creativity, concentration, and coordination.[141] The elite Navy SEAL Team Six, or DEVGRU, actually uses them in training, outfitted with audiovisual inputs to cut the already intensive six-month period of foreign language acquisition to just six weeks.[142]

Other flow states "technologies" are more ancient but just as effective in ways we're beginning to understand.

Yoga, for instance (hatha yoga in particular), is all about harmonizing the body and mind. It systematically challenges the notion of a mind-body split and has been doing so long before "embodied cognition" emerged as an academic field. As researchers like Guy Claxton now emphasize, the body is, above all, an interrelated system of systems. This interrelatedness is a powerful concept, not only explaining connections we've long suspected, like the connection between physical movement and stress reduction, but also surprising connections, like the fantastic fact that striking a dominant pose for two minutes a day can up-regulate testosterone by 20 percent and down-regulate cortisol by 15 percent.[143]

It's no surprise that practitioners in yogic movements frequently experience a sense of energized focus, vibrancy, and peace—the flow state or *dhyana*, to use the yogic parlance. Patanjali's Yoga Sutra lays out specific instructions for attaining this state, first by *pratyahara*, or withdrawing the senses or ignoring distractions, and then by *dharana*, focusing the senses on just one activity or movement.[144]

We can also draw parallels between yoga and other practices, extending to meditation and intense, ecstatic prayer. These modalities appear to be especially effective at fostering selflessness or ego loss. Brain imaging studies carried out by "neurotheologists" have found, for instance, a deactivation of the right parietal lobe during moments of peak spiritual contemplation. This part of the brain is involved in navigation and the perception of distance, and it is based on our awareness of the body's physical boundaries. According to researchers, this deactivation of the right parietal lobe occurs as part of the brain's diversion of energy toward focus. "When this happens, we can no longer distinguish self from other," Andrew Newberg, the lead scientist on the study, says.[145]

Some find the effects of meditation to be strikingly similar to microdosing, while others highlight essential, perhaps complementary, differences. Whereas microdosing enhances energy, sharpness, action, and risk-taking, for example, meditation promotes calm equanimity, emotional grounding, and stillness. Most agree that the efficacy of both modalities at least partially depends on the mindset you bring into them, the optimum being a certain level of calmness, to begin with.[146]

Rhythmic activities such as dancing, drumming, and sex have a similar effect on the brain, synchronizing and channeling neural activity into trance-like focus states. It's interesting to note that song and dance commonly feature in mating rituals, perhaps to showcase an ability to maintain rhythm during intercourse.[147]

Millions of us have experienced moments of what the social scientist Jenny Wade refers to as "transcendent sex." This is the kind of sex that, through a neurochemical cocktail of dopamine, oxytocin, and endorphins, can trigger an almost religious state of selflessness and unity, "identical to those attained by spiritual adepts of all traditions."[148]

It's unfortunate that sex has been so rigidly controlled and suppressed throughout history, not only by religion. For example,

Austrian doctor, sex evangelist, and psychoanalyst Wilhelm Reich's emphasis on the importance of orgasm for overall well-being was heavily stigmatized during his lifetime—even by Sigmund Freud, whose work it influenced. Likewise, pioneering sexologist Alfred Kinsey was derided and obstructed in his efforts to shed light on the vast range of human sexuality.

Nicole Daedone, the founder of OneTaste, is the successor to Kinsey and Reich in many ways—albeit with a far more receptive audience. In true Silicon Valley style, she and her organization have formalized the female orgasm as a Ray Kurzweil-endorsed "technology" for attaining flow states. Known as Orgasmic Meditation (OM), it involves stroking the upper left quadrant of a woman's clitoris to induce a state of neurochemical arousal.

Speaking to a TEDx audience in San Francisco, Daedone predicted a future in which OM would become almost banal, appearing alongside yoga and meditation as a suitable means to induce flow states.[149] As OneTaste's head of marketing Van Vleck put it, "It's like eating breakfast... Instead of a latte, women will have an OM because that's what regulates your body."[150]

Like microdosing, OM is subject to best practice protocols for optimal, or at least reliable, results. The rationale is to create an ideal (non-negotiable) "container" of trust, safety, and efficient reliability—all the more critical with OM or any sexual practice since an orgasm means losing control.

Perhaps nowhere is this more apparent than in the context of BDSM and the sexual expressions of dominance and submission or sadism and masochism. Until as recently as 2010, shortly before the publication of *Fifty Shades of Grey*, the American Psychiatric Association saw BDSM as pathological. Yet, as a 2017 study demonstrated, it's also an exceptionally reliable route into flow states. Following roughly one-hour sessions, practitioners had lower cortisol levels and higher testosterone levels, both essential ingredients of flow.[151] Since BDSM doesn't necessarily involve any rhythmic sexual intercourse, it arguably represents a different modality altogether, channeling focus into the "here and now" through intense stimulation and pointed concentration, and more literally, restricted movement. Nevertheless, even controlling for trust, the risk is undoubtedly still a factor.

The same could be said of extreme sports as well. Big wave surfers, rope-free rock climbers, waterfall kayakers, free divers, and other athletes commonly report an ecstatic sense of timelessness, transcendence, and merging with nature. BASE jumpers, for instance, can enter a "slow-motion" state, even while falling at terminal velocity, allowing them to view their surroundings in intricate detail.

Ultra-endurance athlete Christopher Bergland describes his pursuit of flow as being as much of a curse as a blessing. Although it continually drove him on to greater and greater accomplishments —including a nonstop 135-mile run through Death Valley and a record-breaking 153.76-mile run in just twenty-four hours—not one of them was ultimately enough. "Interestingly," he wrote in *Psychology Today*, "this feeling of total connectedness reminded me of taking psilocybin in high school and was like a drug in and of itself. Needless to say, I became fanatically hooked."[152]

## Cautions

This endless pursuit of flow can, at times, be dangerous. In *Stealing Fire*, Kotler and Wheal give examples of free divers who died from diving too deep. They also relate the story of extreme skier Kristen Ulmer, who courted death worldwide, including on the notorious north face of Aiguille du Midi in Chamonix, France. Like many extreme sports athletes, she was hopelessly hooked on flow, unable to stop pursuing more significant risks despite knowing they'd eventually kill her. Unlike many others, however, she discovered alternative means for achieving the same effect—specifically, through interactive art, group flow, and meditation, avoiding premature death.

Extreme sports are risky, but even meditation can destabilize in unexpected ways. As Vince Horn explained on Third Wave's podcast, the assumption that meditation is always safe and positive is groundless.[153] It's crucial to have support, to be aware of what can happen, and prepare for breakdowns when they occur.

This is why Fadiman's microdosing protocol includes a third day as a return to baseline and also why Kotler and Wheal advise strict control over how often we use ecstatic technology.

The idea that any single modality is essentially superior or inferior to others is problematic but persistent. For instance, some hold that microdosing is inferior to meditation simply because its mastery requires no repetition. This attitude also tends to be prevalent among orthodox religious traditions that have refined and perfected techniques of ecstasy over centuries of practice.

As we continue to study the neurological mechanisms behind the ecstatic state of oneness or unity, a key component of flow states, we may be able to better separate the wheat from the chaff. In addition, we may discover which aspects of traditional or mystical methodologies are necessary for attaining flow states and effectively use scientific data to refine religious praxis.

But all of that is probably beside the point. Humans can access flow states in various ways, but the experience is only valuable if it is a means to an end, not the end itself. The goal is to effect meaningful change in our lives, regardless of our method.

## Practical Considerations for
## Seeking Flow through Microdosing

If you try microdosing with the specific intent of invoking increased creativity and flow states, there are specific tactics you can use to increase your odds of success.

First, carefully consider your choice of substance. While many people find they have nearly identical experiences of microdosing whether they use psilocybin or LSD, several subjective reports suggest that psilocybin leads to more feeling-oriented and self-reflective episodes. LSD, on the other hand, tends to lead to more extroversion, creativity, and focus and can be better for increasing productivity.

In other words, if flow states are your goal, you might have better luck with LSD.

From there, decide on the dose. Taking any amount of psychedelic will increase your ability to engage in potentially productive divergent thinking, the free-flowing, spontaneous, and nonlinear thought pattern that is the exact opposite of the familiar, logic-based "convergent thinking." As a rule of thumb, the higher the dose, the more divergent your thinking tends to be, and the more difficult it is to choose where you focus mental energy.

The extreme means that a 400-microgram dose of LSD can produce highly creative, divergent ways of experiencing the world but would likely result in a limited ability to determine the object of your attention and productively assimilate your observations and thoughts into a practical plan of action. With that in mind, some individuals explicitly seeking to increase their creative output choose to "minidose."

As discussed earlier, a minidose is a dose considered to no longer be genuinely sub-perceptual (all true microdoses are sub-perceptual) but still not as noticeable as a museum dose. Minidosing can be tremendously impactful for creativity and improving abstract reasoning while leaving you with enough control to fully function in normal circumstances and assimilate your divergent thinking into a plan of action.

Finally, be cautious and have a plan in place before you begin.

As we have seen, when you're in a flow state, your impulse control is downregulated; you're more likely to make impulsive decisions. The best way to mitigate this effect is to maintain conscious self-awareness when you microdose and set rules for making decisions. For example, you could make a rule that you will not make any significant decisions while microdosing. Instead, wait twenty-four hours. Then, when a new idea occurs, you can say to yourself, "This sounds like a great idea. Give me a night to sleep on it and we can decide tomorrow."

It's also a good idea to practice microdosing outside the context where you make crucial decisions. For example, take time away from work to experience the effects of microdosing on your body and mind. It will help you develop the self-awareness necessary to sidestep these potential pitfalls to facilitate a more beneficial experience for yourself.

## Want to Go Deeper?

Check out your Microdosing Mastery portal for exclusive resources, articles, and interviews to discover more about the topics from this chapter.

Just go to thethirdwave.co/bonus to access your exclusive book bonuses.

# 12

# Better Leadership through Psychedelics

A s Buckminster Fuller once said: "You never change things by fighting the existing reality. To change something, build a new model that makes the existing model obsolete."

Constant change is the defining characteristic of business in the internet age, bringing exciting new opportunities and significant risks. Legacy business plans can crumble instantly while new models spring up seemingly overnight to take their place. Mobile and internet technology connect people like never before. Many of our objects and devices are hooked into the ever-more extensive web, communicating with one another and collecting and analyzing data that we might not even realize exists.

As the world evolves and we continue to develop new technology at a breathtaking pace, leadership demands are increasing. Leaders need to adapt quickly to new situations and bring a creative, entrepreneurial problem-solving spirit to their endeavors. Microdosing can enhance both abilities. It can also accelerate the developmental process for the next generation of leaders by encouraging honest self-reflection, pushing them toward the pinnacle of their professions. My leadership path and overall character development are closely tied to microdosing—both the modality and the meteoric growth of interest in the topic.

Before starting Third Wave, I had little leadership experience. Most of my decision-making only impacted myself and a handful of English teaching clients from a business perspective. I did not have a team, and I was not speaking publicly about an incendiary topic like psychedelics.

But I yearned for greater responsibility and influence, so I built Third Wave into a credible platform about both microdosing and, generally, the responsible use of psychedelics. As a relatively privileged White male from the United States, I knew it would be easier for me to speak about these substances in a personal, storytelling format that would connect with the mainstream audience I wanted to target. Further, I embodied the "typical" leadership qualities: charismatic, confident, well-spoken, with a propensity to conceptualize new ideas that resonated with other people on a purpose-driven level.

Armed with a passion and a platform, I started Third Wave

and, soon after, organized a microdosing speaking tour across the States and Europe. During the whirlwind year of 2017, I got a crash course in what it meant to become a leader.

What I love about leadership:

- Articulating a vision that speaks to people on a soul-level, catalyzing a desire to contribute to a cause and mission greater than themselves
- Owning my responsibility to speak the truth about uncomfortable topics
- Cultivating and developing skills that directly relate to social intelligence and public speaking
- Empowering team members to take responsibility for their role within an organization and use their purpose and passion to contribute significantly

Challenges in leadership:

- Learning how to deal with direct, personal criticism about a topic of sensitivity; recognizing that I must not personalize criticism, even if it's harsh
- Learning the hard way that I must prioritize self-care or risk burnout and ineffectiveness over the long term

Overall, the lessons I learned about leadership via microdosing in 2017 played a foundational role in my personal development and, thus, the framework laid out in the rest of this chapter.

## New Technologies,
## New Leadership Tools, New Culture

Given the momentous possibilities technology offers, great leaders must develop creative solutions to unexpected issues and problems, quickly turning potential setbacks to their advantage. If your business model isn't disrupting an industry, you can bet that someone will come along soon to disrupt you. Rest on your laurels without striving to be several steps ahead of your competitors, and you are lost. Arriving at the forefront of your field requires mastering new technology and being open to novel ways of accomplishing tasks, taking both short- and long-term needs into account—or seeing with a microscope and a telescope, as a McKinsey leadership forum put it.[154]

How fast do things change? Fast. Entire segments of a market can change in an instant. Consider the effect of Uber and Lyft on the taxicab industry. For decades, the taxicab model was essentially unchallenged for spontaneous, private transport around a city if you didn't have access to a personal car. Municipalities charged high fees to license taxis and imposed heavy regulations, even as a lack of competition allowed the services to stagnate. People learned to live with the status quo.

Until they didn't.

When ride-hailing companies used the power of mobile technology to connect passengers and drivers using an app on their cell phones, suddenly there was a faster, more convenient, and easier way to get a ride. People loved it, and the new models took over a considerable market share nearly overnight. Cities were nearly powerless to stop them, even when they tried to protect traditional taxicabs. That's the kind of massive change entrepreneurial leadership can create.

Sometimes, leaders must respond to changes imposed from the outside as well. Upheaval can come in many forms, from market-shifting events to natural disasters. Shifting alliances, war, migration, an ever-growing human population, and environmental instability all add to the volatile era in which we live. Leadership is most important in these moments of crisis or disturbance; when people feel unsettled, they look to an individual who can guide them through the shifting landscapes and provide clear and insightful decision-making. Navigating uncertainty requires leaders with a vision to help create a better future.

Change happens on a day-to-day level, too. Consider how dramatically the nature of work has changed, rewarding those who can be flexible. For many, particularly those in leadership positions, work is no longer a nine-to-five operation. Instead, people in decision-making roles often need to be accessible at any moment to respond to challenges or emergencies that arise. At the same time, clever entrepreneurs are setting up businesses that can operate for days or months with little maintenance, creating a revenue stream while freeing them to pursue other activities.

That's what I did. I built my online English teaching business with this same goal in mind. Like most young entrepreneurs who read *The 4-Hour Work Week*, I envisioned a future of sitting on remote beaches in Thailand, sipping out of a coconut and soaking in the beautiful rays. While it took slightly longer than expected, my preference for optionality over accumulation created enough freedom that I could have spent my days that way. Instead, I decided to spend the extra time building Third Wave as a premier psychedelic resource.

In early 2017, microdosing hit a cultural inflection point. I took the initiative to co-organize several events across Europe and North America, where I presented public speeches about microdosing. Soon after, I spoke at a major tech conference in Amsterdam called The Next Web. The talk's video went viral and quickly amassed half a million views. This interest in the topic, particularly from the Dutch, inspired my co-founder and me to start Synthesis, a legal psilocybin retreat in the Netherlands. This was in anticipation that psychedelics would be made legal in places like Canada and the United States within a few years. In the Netherlands, we intended to create the blueprint for optimal group psilocybin experiences to help inform an entirely new policy and ecosystem.

Today, Synthesis is intimately involved with developing the legality of psychedelics in Oregon. We've purchased a retreat property in Oregon that will be one of the first centers in the United States to offer legal psilocybin experiences.

Before starting Synthesis, I had done a lot of online education, content publication, and podcasting, but I'd never felt adequately fulfilled by my vocation. Through intention setting and clarity on my North Star, I knew that I craved the human interaction that a place like Synthesis could provide. This clarity fueled my decision to open Synthesis. There was nothing I wanted more than to facilitate and hold space for these experiences. Starting Synthesis was a personally affirming choice that helped lay the foundation for the cultural development of future psychedelic work.

## Changing Needs in an Adapting World

Human ingenuity has created a bittersweet situation: we can be tied to work, in some capacity, for twenty-four hours a day, yet, we can also mold our remote-first work environments to fit our needs and comfort best.[155] Though some jobs require near-constant travel, internet connectivity makes it easy to stay in touch and monitor operations no matter where you are.

Even if you cut your teeth in a traditional workforce and prefer the trappings of a nine-to-five office, you need to be flexible. Not only can a business sink or swim by decisions made (or not) over a night or weekend, but many young employees expect more flexibility in their working conditions and desire more meaning in their work. If you fail to meet those needs, you might find your best employees leaving for someone who does.

No longer can leaders rely on an accepted hierarchy to govern their company's inner workings. Leadership is evolving to be less hierarchical, dominant, and aggressive and more about curating and cultivating space to allow the best people to step in and contribute. In many ways, Uber, though breaking new ground with its services, relied on the old model. They operated in a patriarchal, misogynistic culture that stretched from the executive offices down to reports of harassment allegations against individual drivers.[156] Ultimately, this approach failed, and co-founder Travis Kalanick stepped down as CEO.

The culture of top-down, coercion-based leadership is falling out of style. Outstanding leadership is about more than just disrupting an industry—it's about creating a positive culture where employees are empowered to be their best selves.

Making this change requires managing the ego. Leaders need to be able to set aside the defense of their self-image to take honest feedback from team members—not to mention the millions of voices chiming in from social media—and accept criticism as an opportunity to improve. The feedback leaders receive can be helpful, harsh, and voluminous, and they must be able to take in that input, consider it openly, and move forward with sound decisions. They need to be secure enough to admit when they are wrong but not lose confidence in their vision. Microdosing can help them make this shift.

## Thinking and Feeling

Leaders also need to know when to follow their gut and when to take a more analytic approach to problems. In my work, I refer to this as the balance between "thinking" and "feeling." While analytical thinking is necessary in a world of logic and science, intuition also has its role, particularly in a twenty-first-century world that values relationships.

In my process of building Third Wave, I continue to develop the best ways of balancing these two important ways of being. For example, I have hired team members on several occasions by focusing solely on how their skillsets would allow them to contribute. Determining this fit was task-based—I had to create clear expectations of everyone's tasks.

At other times, the candidate's values have taken center stage in the hiring process. I understand that my feeling and intuition of who the person was and my sense of the values that dictated their work were better predictors of success in the long run. Throughout growing Third Wave, I hired a few people that I knew were not right for the job within a few weeks, not because they lacked the necessary skillsets; they didn't. They looked perfect for the job on paper, but I had a gut feeling that our values and principles weren't in alignment.

It wasn't easy to reverse my original commitment, admit that I had brought on the wrong individuals, and adjust my approach to ensure I hired all subsequent additions with the larger vision front and center.

As a leader, you, too, may find you need to question your default processes; they may be holding you back. Most effective leaders know how to exercise authority, delegate tasks, and manage people.

However, they must also be able to adjust when their tactics aren't working for a particular personality. Such adaptation requires a significant degree of honest self-reflection.

Indeed, author Tony Schwartz in the *Harvard Business Review* suggests the key to twenty-first-century leadership is to "become more wholly human—to develop a wider range of capabilities actively and to understand themselves more deeply."[157] He writes that many of the qualities we associate with good leadership, such as confidence, pragmatism, and decisiveness, can hold us back if we over-rely on them and allow them to become arrogant, unimaginative, and dogmatic. Instead, we need to be able to step past our old bindings and consider exercising qualities that are the opposite of what we have become accustomed to: think humility, imaginativeness, and open-mindedness. Of course, that doesn't mean you should forget the old qualities you used to become a leader in the first place. Instead, you need to cultivate the self-awareness to know when to balance them with what appear to be their opposites.

"The goal is not to find a perfect balance," Schwartz wrote, "but to build a complementary set of strengths, so that we can move gracefully along a spectrum of leadership qualities. Embracing our own complexity makes us more wholly human and gives us additional resources to manage ourselves and others in an increasingly complex world."

Microdosing can help facilitate a flexible balance between productivity, communication, and mental health. By promoting the development of a meta skillset of adaptability, resilience, and creativity, microdosing will be an increasingly potent tool for helping leaders adapt to an uncertain future.

## Emergent and Novel Practice

One function of the world's increasing complexity is the way work is changing. In his book, *The End of Jobs: Money, Meaning and Freedom Without the 9-to-5*, author Taylor Pearson explains the Cynefin framework, a tool developed by Dave Snowden to divide work and management in a way that reflects that change. The framework chops management into four quadrants:

- Simple: when the cause and effect of an issue are clear
- Complicated: when a solution requires more analysis
- Complex: when leaders can't figure out the correct response through experience or education
- Chaotic: when there is no clear relationship between cause and effect, and you need to come up with entirely new ways to move forward

The Cynefin tool includes steps to follow to make progress toward an outcome. The steps are:

- Best practice
- Good practice
- Emergent practice
- Novel practice[158]

As you can see, one of the tried-and-true pillars of good leadership—implementing and following best practices—is only a first step. Best practices are an acceptable way to resolve simple problems. Still, while people whose business concepts are grounded in the twentieth century are concerned with best practices, their entire industries are changing underneath them. Truly ground-breaking leaders function in a realm of complexity that requires them to take an entrepreneurial approach to tackle complex and chaotic issues, driving change in their field instead of struggling to catch up or risking annihilation altogether.

In today's world, simple and even complicated issues are falling by the wayside, subject to mechanization or otherwise becoming obsolete. Yet, true leaders are immersing themselves in the worlds of complex and chaotic problems, developing novel approaches to problem-solving.

Third Wave is an excellent example of an unconventional entre-preneurial initiative. Building the groundwork for a business model around illegal substances is not a "best practices" approach. At first glance, it appears downright stupid. Had I followed best practices in deciding on the first project after my online teaching business, I would have chosen something safe and secure with a clear path to profitability.

Instead, by founding Third Wave, I decided to tackle one of the more complex issues: the prohibition of certain illicit substances with clear medical and psychospiritual benefits for the end-user. At the same time, I balanced my "leap of faith" approach by analyzing several other factors, including the growth in psychedelic research, the legalization of cannabis, and the use of microdosing by the tech world. At that point, I decided to go ahead with the project.

Pearson makes an excellent point about tackling just that sort of complexity. He argues that we have run up against a limit for overall growth and production as a society by focusing on solving simple problems while receiving diminishing returns. That leaves us vulnerable to stagnation and job loss, creating a drag on progress and a drain on resources. Instead, suppose we shift our attention to tackling complex and chaotic problems. In that case, we can surpass our current limits and move into a new economic era that promotes and benefits from the divergent thinking that microdosing can support us.

While you might be reluctant to take the risk of starting your own venture, the potential rewards can far outweigh the drawbacks. In fact, according to Pearson, although most people consider it risky to try new ways of doing things (as I did with Third Wave), entrepreneurship is safer than it's ever been. Because of a cognitive tendency called loss aversion, we understandably fear failure. In other words, we are more swayed by a potential loss than a possible gain. But for most of us, failure in a modern business isn't a high risk. It doesn't mean you'll fall into a life of poverty and humiliation. Usually, a failure is a temporary setback, especially if you have a strong drive to succeed.

Suppose you have a great idea that can make a real difference in the world today. Imagine the vast rewards you could reap if you stayed true to your North Star and weren't dissuaded by the consequences of failure unless they indeed threatened your life or well-being. As we've discussed, microdosing can be an invaluable tool when discovering, naming, evaluating, and pursuing your North Star.

Besides, you can't plan for every eventuality. Sometimes the paths that look sane, sensible, or risk-free can leave you vulnerable to outside forces that could throw all your plans into disarray anyway. If you aren't constantly adapting to stay ahead of looming changes in today's world, you are accumulating silent risk that could build up and harm you when you can least afford it. Pearson uses the example of an accountant who sticks with a steady job, only to be blindsided by a layoff when the company finds a cheaper way to perform the same function. By contrast, an accountant who takes what appears to be a riskier path of starting his own company with greater control of his destiny builds new skills and relationships and has a greater capacity to carve out his role in society. The more entrepreneurial among us don't build up silent risk because they constantly adjust their product or services to meet the current and future needs of the market.

In the modern world, the three motivations shown by research to be most important to humans are money, freedom, and meaning, Pearson writes. When many people think about the profession they intend to follow, they focus on money first and maybe meaning if they are lucky. However, given the technological tools in our hands today, it's easier than ever for intelligent leaders and entrepreneurs to pursue all three goals at once. This can even have an amplifying effect because if you feel like your work is a meaningful choice, not a rote obligation, you are likely to do a better job, thereby increasing the amount of money you earn. "Freedom and meaning aren't something to be put off until after you're rich—they help you get rich," Pearson writes.

"Great work—the kind of work that will create wealth in our lives and the lives of others is not the product of obligation—is the product of freedom," the author continues. "Freedom gives us a longer lever, a better leverage point. By seeking more freedom and building it into our lives, we not only improve our ability to create more material wealth and make more money personally, but we also create more of it in the world at large."

Ultimately, these ideas all come back to Hungarian psychologist Mihaly Csikszentmihalyi's concept of flow. When people become consumed with meeting a goal or overcoming a challenge, immersed in finding new and better ways of completing a task, they feel most happy and fulfilled and, at the same time, create even more valuable work. The adaptability and focus that go hand-in-hand with microdosing perfectly complement this concept.

"As a society, we're paying people more money to do things which create less wealth," writes Pearson. "Yet we're at a point where we can create more wealth and make more money for ourselves and others by pursuing work which forces us to grow in a way we personally find meaningful."

# Tribal Leadership:
## A New Renaissance

Indeed, outstanding leadership can elevate companies and individuals to new levels of excellence by inspiring actions aimed at the common good. In the book *Tribal Leadership*, authors Dave Logan, John King, and Halee Fischer-Wright explain how.[159] Unfortunately, their findings do not touch on microdosing. Still, I've found many qualities and strategies the authors invoke as essential components to unlock the highest levels of success are attributes microdosing can help unleash, such as big-picture vision, empathy, and decisions not based on ego.

This outlook roots in the premise that while the world isn't broken, it can be far better than it is today. While the civilizations of ancient Greece and Rome—and later Europe, during the Renaissance—created the foundations of our modern world, those advances only targeted society's elite, excluding most others.

In *Tribal Leadership*, the authors envision a new renaissance, one that's based on merit alone and not restricted to any location or identity group. Instead, it relies on raising the effectiveness of business cultures, which by and large are bastions of mediocrity, to unleash the potential of the individuals within them.

This model lays out different cultural stages that organizations find themselves in and explores how to accelerate the transition into higher levels of functioning, which will, in turn, attract more people who want to make a real contribution. Culture, in this context, covers both the words that people use to describe themselves, one another, and their work, as well as the structure of relationships and how people connect.

We often think of humanity as grouped into tribes or groups of 150 or fewer people.[160] Those within a particular tribe tend to exhibit certain behaviors, talking and acting in a specific manner. *Tribal Leadership* focuses on culture because the culture of a tribe is stronger than the effect that any one individual can exert. For example, in a business's various departments or groups, we're likely to gain more value from introducing a cultural change across the group than from changing a single person's work. And just as a positive culture can elevate an entire business, an inept or negative one can hold everyone back, even those who would otherwise be high achievers.

"Tribal culture exists in stages, going from undermining to egocentric to history making," the authors write. "Some tribes demand excellence for everyone, and are constantly evolving. Others are content to do the minimum to get by. What makes the difference in performance? Tribal Leaders." If tribal leaders can successfully upgrade their organization's culture, the members (or employees) should respond with their best work. And when everyone is on board and engaged with the work, the tribe or company can produce results that far exceed what any individual, including the leader, could produce alone.

The authors break down tribal culture into five stages:

## Stage One

Stage one groups operate at a survival level, with despairingly hostile people who have no hope of achieving a better life. They estimate that only 2 percent of tribes fall into stage one in the professional world.

## Stage Two

According to the authors, the second stage is larger, making up 25 percent of the employed population. While not as desperate as stage one, negativity still defines it. However, that negativity focuses on individual circumstances, not the world's hopelessness. "People in this cultural stage are passively antagonistic; they cross their arms in judgment yet never really get interested enough to spark any passion," they write. "Their laughter is quietly sarcastic and resigned. The stage two talk is that they've seen it all before and watched it fail."

Notably, even people who have the drive and desire to reach a higher level individually can get bogged down and fail to thrive if all their peers are in a stage two group. Instead, effective leadership would have a better chance to advance if leadership could pull the entire tribe into stage three.

## Stage Three

Here is where most professional cultures in the US are located. They are identifiable by excellence, but more so the excellence of the individual, not the group.

"Within the Stage Three culture, knowledge is power, so people hoard it, from client contacts to gossip about the Company," the authors state. "People at Stage Three have to win, and for them winning is personal. They'll out-work and outthink their competitors on an individual basis." Many companies encourage stage three behavior by measuring the individual's success and creating situations where high performers can shine. Workers compete against one another for rewards like resources and promotions.

You can recognize stage three cultures by group members predominantly using first-person identifiers like "I" and "my," and a scarcity of collaboration, culture-wide innovation, or awareness of shared values.

## Stage Four

By contrast, stage four is a collective of core values and group members working together toward a shared goal. About 22 percent of tribes fall into the stage four classification. There is an enormous opportunity for influential leaders to usher groups from stage three to stage four and release new waves of creativity and success.

The benefits of fostering a stage four culture are myriad, including reducing fear, stress, and friction as collaboration increases and competition is left aside. Morale and general health indicators improve. "The entire tribe shifts from resisting leadership to seeking it out," the authors explain. "Setting and implementing a successful competitive strategy becomes stunningly easy as people's aspirations, knowledge of the market, and creativity are unlocked and shared. Most exciting for us is that people report feeling more alive and having more fun."

The critical question is how leaders can transition a group from stage three to stage four, and how microdosing can play a role in that process. To earn your peers' respect, trust, and buy-in, you need to work on yourself first. Start by making sure you understand the language and customs of people functioning at different stages so that you can meet them at their level and present ideas and concepts in a way that makes sense. At the same time, you need to advance yourself into stage four and bring a core group of people with you to create a center of gravity that positively influences the rest of the tribe.

People have frequently found themselves shaken out of stage three into a more collaborative attitude by significant life changes, such as turning forty and transitioning into middle age or losing a loved one. These events can inspire people to want to give back more to the world instead of focusing only on personal achievement. Notably, a paradigm-shifting experience with moderate doses of psychedelics can have the same result.

When you're ready to move forward in your leadership journey, ask yourself what your ultimate goal is and what you want to accomplish. "As the person sees into her blind spots, she realizes that the ego hit of accomplishment isn't the same as success itself," writes Logan, King, and Fischer-Wright. "Her attention shifts to what's important to her, and almost always, the goal is tribal."

From there, you can start to influence the others around you.

"Instead of speaking for herself and assuming that others will see the logic in her point of view, she begins to listen, to learn about the tribe, and to speak for it," the authors continue. "As all this happens, a subtle but rapid change begins: she accrues respect, loyalty, followers, and an expectation of great things."

This change occurs when you purposefully shift language away from saying "me" and "I" toward words that encompass the goals of the entire group. Language is an essential indicator of culture, and an intentional shift can often lead to a more collaborative mindset. When you start talking more about the common good, it's not that you lose your ego or your drive to succeed. Instead, you learn to direct those things toward the group overall instead of toward individual accolades. You also can observe your ego so you aren't controlled by it. This helps you see and judge yourself objectively, enabling you to make decisions that lead to the best outcome rather than ones that just make you look or feel accomplished.

When you are confident that you are operating in a stage four space yourself, you are ready to flex your leadership and bring your tribe along with you. Remember, the group's core values should be the primary driving force of the organization. Know what values are respected in the group and use language and tactics that reflect them.

To start elevating your colleagues, ask them an escalating series of questions to identify their core values. For example, question someone about what they're proud of, ask why and continue asking why for each response until they stop clearly articulating why something is essential—an indicator that you have reached a core value because it's so ingrained that it can defy expression.

From the outside, you may be able to better articulate this value than the person who holds it. However, once you discover the values of all the people in your tribe and can express them as a shared vision, your leadership will start to take off.

Continue to grow your group into stage four by showing the people around you that networks are more critical to building power than knowledge. Impress upon them that a team working in unison can achieve far more than a single person. Build your team's network by reaching out to people you know who share your values. Create mutually beneficial relationships. Leverage the competitive spirit inherent in stage three but direct it toward other groups or companies, not other individuals.

*Tribal Leadership* also recommends streamlining an approach to building a strategy based on three conversations:

- What we want (outcomes)
- What we have (assets)
- What we will do (behaviors)

"The last epiphany is seeing that the only real goal is the betterment of the tribe," the authors write. "Ironically, as people act to build the tribe, they achieve everything they sought but couldn't achieve at Stage Three: esteem, respect, loyalty, legacy, and enduring success."

Unfortunately, our professional world is defined by stage three behaviors, with people competing to acquire more and more for themselves, regardless of the consequences. Witness banks, pharmaceutical companies, the extraction industry, and others lying, cheating, and generally doing whatever it takes to bring in profits no matter how harmful their practices are to individuals or to the world. Stage three behavior is partially defined by an inability to reflect on itself.

The more companies that start operating at a self-aware, value-driven, stage four level, the better off *everyone* will be as we leave behind antisocial behaviors and strive toward outcomes that transcend the individual's egos.

## Stage Five

This stage represents only 2 percent of professional tribes in the US. "Their language revolves around infinite potential and how the group will make history—not to beat a competitor, but because doing so will make a global impact," the authors write. According to the authors: "This group's mood is 'innocent wonderment,' with people in competition with what's possible, not with another tribe." Stage five groups are the visionaries who change the world.

Most leaders who read this book will see an immediate opportunity to elevate their groups from stage three to stage four. But the genuinely transcendent, those who can harness their collective values into ground-breaking innovation, can create stage five groups and help lead humanity toward a better future.

## Make a Better World

The requirements to succeed as a twenty-first-century entrepreneur —the ability to find creative solutions that address complex or chaotic problems, the capacity to self-reflect honestly and incorporate feedback from several sources in your processes, and the power to tap into a flow state to produce your best, most meaningful work—are things that microdosing supports. Of course, microdosing alone won't make you a great entrepreneur. Still, it does hold the potential to unlock the qualities that leaders need to develop and carry out their visions in a dynamic and fast-changing world.

Successful leaders are those who can form a coherent vision of the future and piece together more accurate models of where the world is going—and how to make it better. For example, as humans recognize that we are sharing a planet with dwindling natural resources, we realize the futility of a zero-sum competitive business model. So instead, more and more companies are moving toward a collaborative, entrepreneurial sharing model.

Society's true leaders will use their skills to create fulfilling ventures while inventing ground-breaking new concepts to transform and improve the whole world.

## Want to Go Deeper?

Check out your Microdosing Mastery portal for exclusive resources, articles, and interviews to discover more about the topics from this chapter.

Just go to thethirdwave.co/bonus to access your exclusive book bonuses.

# Conclusion

F
rom the offices of Silicon Valley to the pages of popular
magazines, the practice of microdosing has become almost
impossible to ignore. As knowledge and awareness develops,
and people experience the tangible benefits of microdosing, the
stigma will fade. All these shifts are helping to legitimize psychedelics in the eyes of mainstream society. With the explosion
of interest in microdosing, we are witnessing the birth of a new
paradigm in psychedelic use.

We are, indeed, in a sea change, riding a powerful Third Wave
that has gathered strength from the research and experimentation
that came before. It has overcome cultural and governmental
backlash, and it is poised to rise to new heights.

Today, the renewed flood of research into psychedelic benefits
combined with microdosing's popularity means that, with diligence and outreach, we can unlock the benefits of psychedelics
for a modern society desperately in need of them. In a world filled
with trauma and upheaval, psychedelics give people a way to heal

the root of their problems without relying on pharmaceutical companies.

Psychedelics can help address an underlying challenge of living in modern society: the lack of human connection. These medicines remind us to be grateful for our friends, family, and the beauty of life. They deepen our empathy and help connect us with nature, spirituality, and the universe. By reducing our egos, we can concentrate on pure creation without feeling shackled by the judgments of others.

Unfortunately, we're not quite there yet. While scientific research offers a promising avenue toward legitimizing the consumption of psychedelics in the eyes of the law and society, it might not be enough to break down the barriers between people and these substances. Facts and research alone aren't enough to sway those of us conditioned to fear and hate psychedelics by decades of propaganda.

The more research and reports that emerge, the more people will feel free to talk openly about these substances. In time, this will increase public acceptance. Unfortunately, psychedelics have been taboo for far too long, subject to misinformation and propaganda, and demonized for political purposes. The prohibition of psychedelics is one of the most significant failures of scientific and political institutions in modern history, a massive setback to the cause of a more just and equitable society.

The stigma is still influential today, discouraging people from even considering psychedelics as anything other than harmful, destructive drugs. In her book, Ayelet Waldman described a friend's reaction when she revealed that she had been microdosing LSD:

> Her face froze. If she had been wearing pearls, she would have clutched them. But, instead, she looked horrified, even disgusted, as if I'd told her that I'd taken up murdering baby seals. Her husband's reaction was only slightly less disturbing. He smiled uncomfortably and changed the subject. I immediately agreed, yes, the antipasto was delicious, and, no, I didn't want any more.
>
> Their reaction launched a series of cascading anxieties. Will I be condemned for doing this? Will people reject me as a nutcase, a crank, a deluded acid freak? Will I lose whatever credibility I have in the world? Will parents not let their children come over to our house anymore, under the misapprehension that I keep drugs in my home? [161]

The prospect of adverse reactions and ostracization could have prevented her from trying the very practice she credited with saving her marriage.

And so, the biggest question of all remains:

"What can we do to move the psychedelic realities into the general culture?"[162]

Here's a few ideas that I'll leave you with:

First, we can engage with people on a cultural level by sharing examples of people using microdosing methods to become happier and more successful, providing a means of connection that also opens the door to a different mindset. In other words, microdosing is an amplifier and accelerator of what is already happening; it does not detach or disconnect us from reality.

And there is reason to believe the landscape will shift. "The information that's increasingly coming out about microdosing makes it more likely that [legalization of LSD] will happen sooner than later," Drug Policy Alliance founder Ethan Nadelmann said during an interview with The Verge.[163] "It's presenting a growing segment of the public with a new perspective on LSD, and it's something that really shatters the images of LSD that people may have in their minds."

Microdosing is a vital tool for initiating conversations about psychedelics on a mainstream level. Conversations like these will start the ball rolling toward legitimizing psychedelics and making them available to people who could benefit from them. This wave is already underway. Meetups and groups dedicated to discussing psychedelics and sharing stories and tips are popping up in cities all around the globe.

It is more crucial than ever to have these cultural conversations. Income inequality is soaring, leaving a large and growing share of wealth and power in the hands of a few families and corporations, exposing billions of others to poverty. Authoritarian governments flex their muscles worldwide, using their power to suppress dissent and harm their weakest and most vulnerable citizens. Necessities like healthcare and education are out of reach for many families. And the climate and environment are on the brink of irrevocable disaster, forcing us to confront whether the planet will continue to be able to sustain human life in the near future.

Psychedelics are not a cure-all for the world's ills; it would be folly to make this claim. But just as psychedelics help individuals come to terms with past traumas and see beyond their egos to find the best path forward, they can play a role in helping the world at large confront traumas and move forward more holistically.

Suppose leaders of large corporations open their minds to goals beyond pulling in the highest possible short-term profits and take on a sense of responsibility for the planet, not just their bottom line. Then, we could see a revolution in the way we conduct commerce.

An entrepreneur's success in microdosing can lead to a virtuous cycle if they funnel wealth back into psychedelic research, leading to greater understanding and destigmatization. And while microdosing alone at nonpsychoactive levels might not be enough to push people toward consciousness-expanding experiments, people who microdose tend to be more likely to try a macrodose to experience its accompanying benefits.

Humanity has a choice to make, perhaps sooner than we think.

Will we continue down a profitable path at all costs, no matter the environmental or human consequences? Or will we cultivate a less destructive way to exist on the planet, live sustainably, and work toward the promotion of the common good?

Dr. Fadiman, the godfather of microdosing, summed up its potential best:

> Of all the results, the most significant, in our estimation, has been the new knowledge gained of the higher processes of the human mind, the framing of new and more productive research questions, and the effect on our understanding of what we can be and what vast potentialities we have still only begun to tap.

# Final Thoughts

*"In theory there is no difference between theory and practice—in practice there is."*

—Yogi Berra

Dear reader,

Thank you so much for your openness and curiosity. Thank you for taking the time and energy to explore a topic on the outer edges of cultural acceptability.

By questioning dogma and investigating what is true for us as individuals, we push the envelope of possibility—we fuel our personal evolution.

That said, there is a very big difference between theory and practice. This is especially true with psychedelics.

Reading about the neurological shifts and possibilities with psychedelics is one thing. It is quite another thing to experience them for yourself.

Microdosing can be very subtle.

Your mind becomes slippery, and it is surprisingly easy to miss your significant insights and growth opportunities.

This is where an experienced coach can make a huge difference. They keep you accountable to your process. They can pick up on the key details you may have missed. They help you dial in your protocol so you get actual value and long-term shifts instead of just a fleeting experience.

A coach helps you get what you want most from microdosing.

Whether you are a total beginner or have years of experience, there is always something to be learned.

There is always room to get better.

If that sounds useful to you, I invite you to check out Third Wave's private coaching program at: thethirdwave.co/microdosing -coaching/

Our coaches go through a rigorous training process with some of the best teachers in the world. They are highly effective coaches, inspired, compassionate humans, and know the psychedelic experience inside and out.

They can help you master the skill of psychedelics to support your healing, fuel your goals, and catalyze your personal evolution.

Or, if you are interested in pursuing psychedelic coaching professionally, I invite you to check out our Coaching Certification Program.

The program draws on both traditional and modern approaches to psychedelic medicines and combines them with modern coaching methodologies, neuroscience, breathwork, and several other modalities.

In short, you learn to master the skill of psychedelics to transform your own life. We then show you how to teach others that same skill.

For more information, go to:
thethirdwave.co/coaching-certification/.

# Endnotes

1   Tracy L. Barnett, "Mining and Poaching Threatens 15,000-Year-Old Peyote
    Tradition in Mexico," *DoubleBlind*, November 24, 2021, https://doubleblind
    mag.com/mining-and-poaching-threatens-15000-year-old-peyote-tradition-in
    -mexico/.

2   Erin Blakemore, "Ancient Hallucinogens Found in 1,000-Year-Old Shamanic
    Pouch," *National Geographic*, May 6, 2019, https://www.nationalgeographic.com
    /culture/article/ancient-hallucinogens-oldest-ayahuasca-found-shaman-pouch.

3   Wesley Thoricatha, "The Search for Soma, the Ancient Indian Psychedelic,"
    *Psychedelic Times,* November 4, 2015, https://psychedelictimes.com/the-search
    -for-soma-the-ancient-indian-psychedelic/.

4   Brian C. Muraresku, *The Immortality Key: The Secret History of the Religion with
    No Name* (New York: St. Martin's Press, 2020).

5   Olivia Goldhill, "The Foundation of Western Philosophy is Probably Rooted in
    Psychedelics," *Quartz*, August 12, 2017, https://qz.com/1051128/the
    -philosophical-argument-that-every-smart-person-should-do-psychedelics/.

6   Muraresku, *The Immortality Key*.

7   R. R. Griffiths et al., "Psilocybin can Occasion Mystical-Type Experiences
    Having Substantial and Sustained Personal Meaning and Spiritual Significance,"
    *Psychopharmacology* 187, no. 3 (July 7, 2006): 268–83, https://doi.org/10.1007
    /s00213-006-0457-5; Ben Cheng et al., "Job Satisfaction: 2014 Edition,"
    The Conference Board, June 18, 2014, https://www.conference-board.org
    /research/job-satisfaction/job-satisfaction-2014.

8   Tom LoBianco, "Report: Aide Says Nixon's War on Drugs Targeted Blacks,
    Hippies," *CNN*, March 24, 2016, https://www.cnn.com/2016/03/23/politics
    /john-ehrlichman-richard-nixon-drug-war-blacks-hippie/index.html.

9   Marcy C. McCall, "In Search of Yoga: Research Trends in a Western Medical Database," *International Journal of Yoga* 7, no. 1 (January–June 2014): 4–8, https://doi.org/10.4103%2F0973-6131.123470; Jeff Wilson, *Mindful America: The Mutual Transformation of Buddhist Meditation and American Culture* (New York: Oxford University Press, 2014).

10  Wesley Lowery, "Introducing the Real Will Smith," *GQ*, September 27, 2021, https://www.gq.com/story/will-smith-november-cover-profile.

11  David Marchese, "Brad Pitt on the Kind of Leading Man He Doesn't Want to Be," *The New York Times Magazine*, December 9, 2019, https://www.nytimes.com/interactive/2019/12/09/magazine/brad-pitt-interview.html.

12  Olivia Solon, "Under Pressure, Silicon Valley Workers Turn to LSD Microdosing," *Wired*, August 24, 2016, https://www.wired.co.uk/article/lsd-microdosing-drugs-silicon-valley.

13  Terence McKenna, *Food of the Gods: The Search for the Original Tree of Knowledge—A Radical History of Plants, Drugs, and Human Evolution* (New York: Bantam Books, 1992).

14  Michael Horowitz, "An Interview with Albert Hofmann," *High Times*, 1976, https://erowid.org/culture/characters/hofmann_albert/hofmann_albert_interview1.pdf.

15  Stephie Grob Plante, "LSD Microdoses Make People Feel Sharper, and Scientists Want to Know How," The Verge, April 24, 2017, https://www.theverge.com/2017/4/24/15403644/microdosing-lsd-acid-productivity-benefits-brain-studies.

16  Willis W. Harman et al., "Psychedelic Agents in Creative Problem-Solving: A Pilot Study," *Psychological Reports* 19, no. 1 (August 1, 1966): 211–27, https://doi.org/10.2466%2Fpr0.1966.19.1.211.

17  James Fadiman, *The Psychedelic Explorer's Guide: Safe, Therapeutic, and Sacred Journeys* (Rochester, VT: Park Street Press, 2011).

18  Josh Dean, "Micro-Dosing: The Drug Habit Your Boss Is Gonna Love," *GQ*, January 4, 2017, https://www.gq.com/story/micro-dosing-lsd.

19  Matthew Korfhage, "We're Entering a New Golden Age of Psychedelics, and Portland is Leading the Way," *Willamette Week*, April 18, 2017, https://www.wweek.com/culture/2017/04/18/can-lsd-make-you-better-at-your-job-the-guy-in-the-cubicle-next-to-you-might-be-trying-it/.

20  Nathan Heller, "How Ayelet Waldman Found a Calmer Life on Tiny Doses of LSD," *The New Yorker*, January 12, 2017, https://www.newyorker.com/culture /persons-of-interest/how-ayelet-waldman-found-a-calmer-life-on-tiny-doses -of-lsd.

21  Maria Gallucci, "Researchers Want to Know the Effects of Taking Small Doses of LSD to Self-Medicate," *Mashable*, May 9, 2017, https://mashable.com/article /lsd-microdosing-scientific-study; Emma Hogan, "Turn On, Tune In, Drop By the Office," *The Economist*, August 1, 2017, https://www.1843magazine.com /features/turn-on-tune-in-drop-by-the-office; Craig K. Comstock, "Psychedelics and Normality," *HuffPost*, July 25, 2017, http://www.huffingtonpost.com/entry /psychedelics-and-normality_us_5977a1dae4b01cf1c4bb73dc; Miss Rosen, "Better Living Through Microdosing," *Mandatory*, May 5, 2017, https://www .mandatory.com/living/1258901-better-living-microdosing; Korfhage, "We're Entering a New Golden Age of Psychedelics"; Catrin Nye, "Microdosing: The People Taking LSD with Their Breakfast," *BBC News*, April 10, 2017, http://www.bbc.co.uk/news/health-39516345.

22  Jill Petzinger, "How Microdosing Psychedelics Like LSD Could Boost Your Leadership Skills," *Quartz*, July 22, 2017, https://qz.com/1036444/lsd-in-microdoses -can-make-you-a-better-manager-says-paul-austin-of-the-third-wave/.

23  Stephie Grob Plante, "Meet the World's First Online LSD Microdosing Coach," *Rolling Stone*, September 7, 2017, https://www.rollingstone.com/culture/culture -features/meet-the-worlds-first-online-lsd-microdosing-coach-195817/.

24  Colleen Hagerty, "The 'Psychedelics Coach' With Drug-Fuelled Career Advice," *BBC*, January 6, 2020, https://www.bbc.com/worklife/article/20200106-can -drugs-help-you-choose-a-new-career.

25  "Microdosing: Sub-Threshold Dosing of Psychedelic Drugs for Self-Improvement, Therapy or Well-Being," r/microdosing, Reddit, accessed August 10, 2022, https://www.reddit.com/r/microdosing/.

26  u/marc1411, "Random Observations 7 Weeks in MD Mushrooms," r/microdosing, Reddit, April 30, 2017, https://www.reddit.com/r/microdosing/comments/68 fnr0/random_observations_7_weeks_in_md_mushrooms/.

27  u/maths-n-drugs, "Micro-Dosing and Mathematics," r/microdosing, Reddit, April 24, 2017, https://www.reddit.com/r/microdosing/comments/67ctik /microdosing_and_mathematics/.

28  "About Microdosing," Beckley Foundation, accessed August 10, 2022, http://beckleyfoundation.org/microdosing-lsd/.

29  Vince Polito and Richard J. Stevenson, "A Systematic Study of Microdosing Psychedelics," *PLoS ONE* 14, no. 2 (February 6, 2019), https://doi.org/10.1371 /journal.pone.0211023.

30  Jason Koebler, "A Brief History of Microdosing," *Vice*, November 24, 2015, https:// motherboard.vice.com/en_us/article/gv5p5y/a-brief-history-of-microdosing.

31  Petter Grahl Johnstad, "Powerful Substances in Tiny Amounts: An Interview Study of Psychedelic Microdosing," *Nordic Studies on Alcohol and Drugs* 35, no. 1 (February 2018): 39–51, https://doi.org/10.1177/1455072517753339.

32  Thomas Anderson et al., "Psychedelic Microdosing Benefits and Challenges: An Empirical Codebook," *Harm Reduction Journal* 16, no. 1 (July 10, 2019): 43, https://doi.org/10.1186/s12954-019-0308-4.

33  Polito and Stevenson, "A Systematic Study of Microdosing Psychedelics," *PLoS ONE*.

34  Michael Pollan, "The Trip Treatment," *The New Yorker*, February 2, 2015, http://www.newyorker.com/magazine/2015/02/09/trip-treatment.

35  Rebecca Coffey, "Microdosing, and the Gentrification of Psychedelic Culture. A Conversation With Sociologist Dimitrios Liokaftos," *Forbes*, June 29, 2021, https://www.forbes.com/sites/rebeccacoffey/2021/06/29/microdosing-and-the -gentrification-of-psychedelic-culture-a-conversation-with-sociologist-dimitrios -liokaftos/?sh=68ed7beffac7.

36  David Jay Brown, *The New Science of Psychedelics: At the Nexus of Culture, Conscious- ness, and Spirituality* (Rochester, VT: Park Street Press, 2013).

37  Janet Chang, "A Year-Long Microdosing Experiment," 2017, in *The Third Wave*, podcast, 1:04:42, https://thethirdwave.co/podcast/episode-30-janet-chang/.

38  Janet L. Chang, "How One Year of Microdosing Psilocybin Helped My Career, Relationships, and Happiness," *Better Humans*, September 21, 2017, https://betterhumans.coach.me/how-one-year-of-microdosing-helped-my -career-relationships-and-happiness-715dbccdfae4.

39  Fadiman, *The Psychedelic Explorer's Guide*.

40  Steliana Yanakieva et al., "The Effects of Microdose LSD on Time Perception: A Randomised, Double-Blind, Placebo-Controlled Trial," *Psychopharmacology* 236 (November 26, 2018): 1159–70, https://doi.org/10.1007/s00213-018-5119-x.

41  Rosalind Stone, "'Nobody Knows I'm a Mermaid': There's More to Microdosing than Productivity," *Third Wave* (blog), June 23, 2017, https://thethirdwave.co /microdosing-life-lessons/.

42  Anya K. Bershad et al., "Acute Subjective and Behavioral Effects of Microdoses of Lysergic Acid Diethylamide in Healthy Human Volunteers," *Biological Psychiatry* 86, no. 10 (November 15, 2019): 792–800, https://doi.org/10.1016/j.biopsych.2019.05.019.

43  Lennard J. Davis, "Five Reasons to Think Twice about SSRIs," *Psychology Today*, January 7, 2010, https://www.psychologytoday.com/blog/obsessively-yours/201001/five-reasons-not-take-ssris.

44  Roni Caryn Rabin, "Mental Health: Deficiencies in Treatment of Depression," *The New York Times,* January 8, 2010, http://www.nytimes.com/2010/01/12/health/12ment.html?ref=health.

45  Shamsah B. Sonawalla and Jerrold F. Rosenbaum, "Placebo Response in Depression," *Dialogues in Clinical* Neuroscience 4, no. 1 (March 2022): 105–13, https://doi.org/10.31887%2FDCNS.2002.4.1%2Fssonawalla.

46  "23 Best Psychological Thriller Books That Will Mess with Your Head," *Discovery* (blog), Reedsy, December 21, 2018, https://reedsy.com/discovery/blog/psychological-thriller-books.

47  Robin L. Carhart-Harris, "Serotonin, Psychedelics and Psychiatry," *World Psychiatry* 17, no. 3 (October 2018): 358–59, https://doi.org/10.1002/wps.20555.

48  Fadiman, *The Psychedelic Explorer's Guide.*

49  James Fadiman and Sophia Korb, "James Fadiman & Sophia Korb: Microdosing—The Phenomenon, Research Results & Startling Surprises," MAPS, April 26, 2017, YouTube video, 1:02:05, https://www.youtube.com/watch?v=JBgKRyRCVFM.

50  Joseph M. Rootman et al., "Adults Who Microdose Psychedelics Report Health Related Motivations and Lower Levels of Anxiety and Depression Compared to Non-Microdosers," *Scientific Reports* 11 (November 28, 2021), https://doi.org/10.1038/s41598-021-01811-4.

51  Andrew Leonard, "How LSD Microdosing Became the Hot New Business Trip," *Rolling Stone,* November 20, 2015, https://www.rollingstone.com/culture/culture-news/how-lsd-microdosing-became-the-hot-new-business-trip-64961/.

52  Korfhage, "We're Entering a New Golden Age of Psychedelics."

53  Fadiman and Korb, "Microdosing," YouTube video.

54  Hogan, "Turn On, Tune In."

55  u/microtrooper, "7 Months Microdosing. Full Report, Experiences and Thoughts," r/microdosing, Reddit, June 6, 2015, https://www.reddit.com/r/microdosing /comments/38sef1/7_months_microdosing_full_report_experiences_and/.

56  "Microdosing Revisited, Effects on Athletic Performance/Intense Cardio?" r/microdosing, Reddit, April 24, 2017, https://www.reddit.com/r/microdosing /comments/67bsf4/microdosing_revisited_effects_on_athletic/; u/Lsdusaa, "I Decided to Start Sprinting/Running on LSD," r/LSD, Reddit, October 2, 2014, https://www.reddit.com/r/LSD/comments/2i353x/i_decided_to_start _sprintingrunning_on_lsd/.

57  Fadiman, *The Psychedelic Explorer's Guide.*

58  Erica Avey, "Do Psychedelics Alter the Menstrual Cycle?" *DoubleBlind*, March 17, 2021, https://doubleblindmag.com/periods-and-psychedelics/.

59  Johannes G. Ramaekers et al., "A Low Dose of Lysergic Acid Diethylamide Decreases Pain Perception in Healthy Volunteers," *Journal of Psychopharmacology* 35, no. 4 (April 2021): 398–405, https://doi.org/10.1177/0269881120940937.

60  James Fadiman, "The Genesis of Microdosing: Creativity, Problem-Solving, and Other Feats of Mental Magic," February 28, 2021, in *The Third Wave*, podcast, 1:26:41, https://thethirdwave.co/podcast/episode-116-james-fadiman/.

61  Paul Austin, "LSD vs. Psilocybin: What's the Difference?" Third Wave, July 23, 2021, YouTube video, 4:28, https://www.youtube.com/watch?v=cOx_-4ab3os.

62  "Struggling with Depression in Silicon Valley," Mental Health Therapy News, *The Panelist*, accessed August 12, 2022, https://thepanelist.net/struggling-with -depression-in-silicon-valley/.

63  "Silicon Valley's Secret," *Mostly Human with Laurie Segall*, CNN, directed by Roxy Hunt, 2017, http://money.cnn.com/mostly-human/silicon-valleys-secret/.

64  Ayelet Waldman, *A Really Good Day: How Microdosing Made a Mega Difference in My Mood, My Marriage, and My Life* (New York: Knopf, 2017).

65  Ayelet Waldman, "Microdosing for a Really Good Day," March 8, 2017, in *The Third Wave*, podcast, 45:53, https://thethirdwave.co/ayelet-waldman-really -good-day/.

66  Alex Williams, "How LSD Saved One Woman's Marriage," *The New York Times*, January 7, 2017, https://www.nytimes.com/2017/01/07/style/microdosing-lsd -ayelet-waldman-michael-chabon-marriage.html.

67  Rachel Cooke, "How Dropping Acid Saved My Life," *The Guardian*, January 7, 2017, https://www.theguardian.com/global/2017/jan/08/how-dropping-acid -saved-my-life-ayelet-waldman-books-depression.

68  "LSD in 'Microdoses' Can Improve Mood, Productivity, Some Claim," *Brain Power TODAY*, Today, February 8, 2017, http://www.today.com/video/lsd-in -microdoses-can-improve-mood-productivity-some-claim-872494659553.

69  Heller, "How Ayelet Waldman Found a Calmer Life."

70  Nadia R. P. W. Hutten et al., "Low Doses of LSD Acutely Increase BDNF Blood Plasma Levels in Healthy Volunteers," *ACS Pharmacology & Translational Science* 4, no. 2 (2021): 461–66, https://doi.org/10.1021/acsptsci.0c00099.

71  Waldman, *A Really Good Day*.

72  Ling-Xiao Shao et al., "Psilocybin Induces Rapid and Persistent Growth of Dendritic Spines in Frontal Cortex in Vivo," *Neuron* 109, no. 16 (August 18, 2021): 2535–44. E4, https://doi.org/10.1016/j.neuron.2021.06.008.

73  Marc Dingman, "Know Your Brain: Default Mode Network," *Neuroscientifically Challenged* (blog), accessed August 12, 2022, http://www.neuroscientifically challenged.com/blog/know-your-brain-default-mode-network.

74  Andrea Anderson, "LSD May Chip Away at the Brain's 'Sense of Self' Network," *Scientific American*, April 13, 2016, https://www.scientificamerican.com/article /lsd-may-chip-away-at-the-brain-s-sense-of-self-network/.

75  Milan Scheidegger, "Milan Scheidegger: Psilocybin & Mindfulness in a Meditation Retreat Setting," MAPS, April 26, 2017, YouTube video, 31:59, https://www.youtube.com/watch?v=LZ9Vp4Hz5IU&list=PL4F0vNNTozFS w5gRe_zVTAvNIwjYD_AIU.

76  Vanja Palmers, "Meditation and Psychedelics," *MAPS* 11, no. 2 (Fall 2001): 43–44, http://www.maps.org/news-letters/v11n2/11243pal.html.

77  Peter Gasser et al., "Safety and Efficacy of Lysergic Acid Diethylamide-Assisted Psychotherapy for Anxiety Associated with Life-Threatening Diseases," *The Journal of Nervous and Mental Disease* 202, no. 7 (2014): 513–20, https://doi.org/10.1097%2FNMD.0000000000000113.

78  Teri S. Krebs and Pål-Ørjan Johansen, "Lysergic Acid Diethylamide (LSD) for Alcoholism: Meta-Analysis of Randomized Controlled Trials," *Journal of Psychopharmacology* 26, no. 7 (July 1, 2012): 994–1002, https://doi.org/10 .1177%2F0269881112439253.

79 Robin L. Carhart-Harris et al., "Neural Correlates of the LSD Experience Revealed by Multimodal Neuroimaging," *Proceedings of the National Academy of Sciences* 113, no. 17 (April 11, 2016): 4853–58, https://doi.org/10.1073/pnas.1518377113.

80 Kate Wighton, "The Brain on LSD Revealed: First Scans Show How the Drug Affects the Brain," *Imperial College London News*, April 11, 2016, http://www3.imperial.ac.uk/newsandeventspggrp/imperialcollege/news summary/news_11-4-2016-17-21-2.

81 Francisco A. Moreno et al., "Safety, Tolerability, and Efficacy of Psilocybin in 9 Patients with Obsessive-Compulsive Disorder," *The Journal of Clinical Psychiatry* 67, no. 11 (November 2006): 1735–40, https://doi.org/10.4088/jcp.v67n1110.

82 Briony J. Catlow et al., "Effects of Psilocybin on Hippocampal Neurogenesis and Extinction of Trace Fear Conditioning," *Experimental Brain Research* 228, no. 4 (August 2013): 481–91, https://doi.org/10.1007/s00221-013-3579-0.

83 Robin L. Carhart-Harris et al., "Psilocybin with Psychological Support for Treatment-Resistant Depression: An Open-Label Feasibility Study," *Lancet Psychiatry* 3, no. 7 (July 1, 2016): 619–27, https://doi.org/10.1016/S2215-0366(16)30065-7.

84 Charles S. Grob et al., "Pilot Study of Psilocybin Treatment for Anxiety in Patients with Advanced-Stage Cancer," *Archives of General Psychiatry* 68, no. 1 (January 2011): 71–78, https://doi.org/10.1001/archgenpsychiatry.2010.116.

85 Vanessa McMains, "Hallucinogenic Drug Found in 'Magic Mushrooms' Eases Depression, Anxiety in People with Life-Threatening Cancer," *Hub*, Johns Hopkins University, November 30, 2016, https://hub.jhu.edu/2016/12/01/hallucinogen-treats-cancer-depression-anxiety/.

86 Stephen Ross et al., "Rapid and Sustained Symptom Reduction Following Psilocybin Treatment for Anxiety and Depression in Patients with Life-Threatening Cancer: A Randomized Controlled Trial," *Journal of Psychopharmacology* 30, no. 12 (November 30, 2016): 1165–80, https://doi.org/10.1177/0269881116675512.

87 Annie Levy, "Annie Levy—Psilocybin Study Participant," Heffter Research Institute, October 26, 2014, YouTube video, 7:00, https://www.youtube.com/watch?v=xYhtXI4Prpo&feature=youtu.be.

88 Laurie Kershman, "Kershman: Benefits from the Johns Hopkins Psilocybin Study," Heffter Research Institute, March 14, 2014, YouTube video, 13:15, https://www.youtube.com/watch?v=OefUwXIKj90&feature=youtu.be.

89  G. Petri et al., "Homological Scaffolds of Brain Functional Networks," *Journal of the Royal Society Interface* 11, no. 101 (December 6, 2014), https://doi.org/10.1098/rsif.2014.0873.

90  Franca Davenport, "New Study Discovers Biological Basis for Magic Mushroom 'Mind Expansion,'" *Imperial College London News*, July 3, 2014, http://www3.imperial.ac.uk/newsandeventspggrp/imperialcollege/news summary/news_2-7-2014-18-11-12.

91  "Tripping Up: The Real Danger of Microdosing with LSD," *New Scientist*, June 14, 2017, https://www.newscientist.com/article/mg23431303-300-tripping -up-the-real-danger-of-microdosing-with-lsd/.

92  Zachary Siegel, "LSD's Health Benefits Convince Norway to Relax Punishment for Possession," *Vice*, October 6, 2017, https://tonic.vice.com/en_us/article/ne7m 4m/lsds-health-benefits-norway-possession.

93  "Microdosing LSD and Its Research Potential," *Heffter Blog*, Heffter Research Institute, August 17, 2021, http://heffter.org/microdosing-lsd-research-potential/.

94  Fadiman and Korb, "Microdosing," YouTube video.

95  Alex Brewer, "12 Medications That Can Lower the Seizure Threshold," GoodRx Health, April 20, 2022, https://www.goodrx.com/healthcare-access/medication -education/drugs-that-lower-seizure-threshold.

96  "Iboga," RxList, last modified June 11, 2021, https://www.rxlist.com/iboga /supplements.htm.

97  Paul Austin, "Why Set and Setting Matters for Microdosing," *Third Wave* (blog), September 15, 2020, https://thethirdwave.co/why-set-and-setting-matters-for -microdosing/#.

98  Ryan O'Hare, "Citizen Scientists Show Placebo Effect May Explain Benefits of Microdosing," *Imperial College London News*, March 2, 2021, https://www .imperial.ac.uk/news/216134/citizen-scientists-show-placebo-effect-explain/.

99  "Is Microdosing Just a Placebo?" *Third Wave* (blog), June 4, 2017, https:// thethirdwave.co/microdosing-placebo/.

100  Yandiel Muniz, "Designer Drugs and the Federal Analog Act," *FIU Law Review* (blog), FIU Law, March 11, 2017, https://law.fiu.edu/designer-drugs -federal-analog-act/; Erowid, "Introduction to the Federal Controlled Substance Analogue Act," *The Vaults of Erowid* (blog), January 2001, https://www.erowid .org/psychoactives/law/analog/analog_info1.shtml.

101 "Mushroom Grow Kit," Third Wave, accessed September 7, 2022, https://the thirdwave.co/sp/mushroom-grow-kit/.

102 Adam Gottlieb, *Peyote and Other Psychoactive Cacti* (Berkeley: Ronin Publishing, 1977).

103 Caine Barlow, "Growing San Pedro Cactus: A Complete How-To," *Third Wave* (blog), December 8, 2021, https://thethirdwave.co/growing-san-pedro-cactus/.

104 This is possibly ideal if you're a first-timer and work weekdays, since you'll have the day off to comfortably test the immediate effects and the following day to observe the residual effects in the workplace.

105 Kyle Dow, "Microdosing Psilocybin Mushrooms with the Stamets Stack," *Third Wave* (blog), November 19, 2019, https://thethirdwave.co/microdosing -psilocybin-mushrooms-stamets-stack/.

106 Fadiman and Korb, "Microdosing," YouTube video.

107 Deep breathing means inhaling into the diaphragm, or the abdomen, rather than the chest.

108 Michael Craig Miller, "In Praise of Gratitude," *Harvard Health Blog*, Harvard Health Publishing, November 21, 2012, https://www.health.harvard.edu/blog /in-praise-of-gratitude-201211215561.

109 u/Bancopuma, "Iboga Microdosing Guide," Other Entheogens, DMT-Nexus, December 27, 2013, https://www.dmt-nexus.me/forum/default.aspx?g=posts &t=52279.

110 At least in the case of LSD and psilocybin. Some other psychedelics may need longer.

111 Erin Ginder-Shaw, "Learn About Cutting-Edge Microdosing Research from Dr. Jim Fadiman," *Third Wave* (blog), May 3, 2017, https://thethirdwave.co /microdosing-psychedelic-science-2017/.

112 Rotem Petranker et al., "Microdosing Psychedelics: Subjective Benefits and Challenges, Substance Testing Behavior, and the Relevance of Intention," *Journal of Psychopharmacology* 36, no. 1 (2022): 85–96, https://doi.org/10.11 77%2F0269881120953994.

113 Rootman et al., "Adults Who Microdose Psychedelics."

114 Gregory Frederick Ferenstein, "Third Wave Lab: A Case Report on Preventative Psilocybin Use," The Lab, Third Wave, accessed August 15, 2022, https:// thethirdwave.co/lab/preventative-psilocybin-use/.

115   u/WintersTwin, "Diminished Alcohol Craving!" r/microdosing, Reddit, September 21, 2017, https://www.reddit.com/r/microdosing/comments/71i1c8 /diminished_alcohol_craving/.

116   "'Magic Mushrooms' Help Longtime Smokers Quit," Johns Hopkins Medicine, September 11, 2014, https://www.hopkinsmedicine.org/news/media/releases /magic_mushrooms_help_longtime_smokers_quit.

117   Gregory Frederick Ferenstein and Liz Zhou, "Case Study: Microdosing to Cut Stress-Smoking and Caffeine," The Lab, Third Wave, accessed August 15, 2022, https://thethirdwave.co/lab/microdosing-to-cut-stress-smoking-and-caffeine/.

118   Erica Fink, "When Silicon Valley Takes LSD," *CNN Business*, January 25, 2015, http://money.cnn.com/2015/01/25/technology/lsd-psychedelics-silicon-valley/.

119   Fink, "When Silicon Valley Takes LSD."

120   Hogan, "Turn On, Tune In."

121   Wendy M. Grossman, "Did the Use of Psychedelics Lead to a Computer Revolution?" *The Guardian*, September 6, 2011, https://www.theguardian.com /commentisfree/2011/sep/06/psychedelics-computer-revolution-lsd.

122   John Markoff, *What the Dormouse Said: How the Sixties Counterculture Shaped the Personal Computer Industry* (New York: Viking Penguin, 2005).

123   Nellie Bowles, "At HBO's 'Silicon Valley' Premier, Elon Musk Has Some Notes," *Vox*, April 3, 2014, https://www.recode.net/2014/4/3/11625260/at-hbos-silicon -valley-premiere-elon-musk-is-pissed.

124   Drew Olanoff, "Google CEO Larry Page Shares His Philosophy at I/O: 'We Should Be Building Great Things That Don't Exist,'" *Tech Crunch*, May 15, 2013, https://techcrunch.com/2013/05/15/google-ceo-larry-page-takes-the -stage-at-ceo-to-wrap-up-the-io-keynote/.

125   James Oroc, "Psychedelics and Extreme Sports," *MAPS Bulletin* 21, no. 1 (Spring 2011): 25–29, http://www.maps.org/news-letters/v21n1/v21n1-25to29.pdf.

126   Tim Ferriss, "Are Psychedelic Drugs the Next Medical Breakthrough? (#104)" September 14, 2015, in *The Tim Ferris Show*, podcast, 1:47:07, http://tim.blog /2015/09/14/are-psychedelic-drugs-the-next-medical-breakthrough/.

127   Tim Ferriss, "The Psychedelic Explorer's Guide—Risks, Micro-Dosing, Ibogaine, and More (#66)," March 21, 2015, in *The Tim Ferriss Show*, podcast, 1:36:54, http://tim.blog/2015/03/21/james-fadiman/.

128   Joe Rogan, "Joe Rogan on Micro-Dosing Psilocybin," JRE Clips, April 18, 2017, YouTube video, 7:21, https://www.youtube.com/watch?v=pUWaZ_wxhhg.

129   Steven Kotler and Jamie Wheal, *Stealing Fire: How Silicon Valley, the Navy SEALs, and Maverick Scientists Are Revolutionizing the Way We Live and Work* (New York: Dey Street Books, 2017).

130   Mihaly Csikszentmihalyi, *Flow: The Psychology of Optimal Experience* (New York: Harper & Row, 1990).

131   Fadiman, *The Psychedelic Explorer's Guide.*

132   Baynard Woods, "Can Very Small Doses of LSD Make You a Better Worker? I Decided to Try It," *Vox*, March 2, 2016, http://www.vox.com/2016/3/2/1111 5974/lsd-internet-addiction.

133   Katie Herzog, "Adventures in Microdosing," *The Stranger*, March 8, 2017, http://www.thestranger.com/features/2017/03/08/25008382/adventures-in -microdosing.

134   Harman et al., "Psychedelic Agents in Creative Problem-Solving."

135   Peter G. Stafford and Bonnie Helen Golightly, *LSD: The Problem-Solving Psychedelic* (New York: Award Books, 1967).

136   Anna Ermakova and Rosalind Stone, "Ayahuasca and Creativity: The Amazonian Plant Brew Improves Divergent Thinking," Beckley Foundation, July 29, 2016, http://beckleyfoundation.org/2016/07/29/ayahuasca-and-creativity/.

137   Neiloufar Family et al., "Semantic Activation in LSD: Evidence from Picture Naming," *Language, Cognition and Neuroscience* 31, no. 10 (August 11, 2016): 1320–27, https://doi.org/10.1080/23273798.2016.1217030.

138   "LSD and Associative Thinking," *The Psychedelic Scientist* (blog), October 1, 2016, https://thepsychedelicscientist.com/2016/10/01/lsd-and-associative-thinking/.

139   Ian Sample, "LSD's Impact on the Brain Revealed in Groundbreaking Images," *The Guardian*, April 11, 2016, https://www.theguardian.com/science/2016/apr /11/lsd-impact-brain-revealed-groundbreaking-images.

140   Kotler and Wheal, *Stealing Fire.*

141   Shelly Fan, "Floating Away: The Science of Sensory Deprivation Therapy," *Discover*, April 4, 2014, https://www.discovermagazine.com/health/floating -away-the-science-of-sensory-deprivation-therapy.

142   Mark Divine, "Jamie Wheal Talks About the Flow State," February 15, 2017, in *Unbeatable Mind*, podcast, 54:46, http://unbeatablemind.com/jamie-wheal/.

143   Amy Cuddy, "Your Body Language May Shape Who You Are," 2012, TED Talk, video, 20:46, https://www.ted.com/talks/amy_cuddy_your_body_language _shapes_who_you_are.

144   Esther Ekhart, "The 'Flow State' and How to Get There," *EkhartYoga* (blog), accessed August 15, 2022, https://www.ekhartyoga.com/articles/the-flow-state -and-how-to-get-there.

145   Kotler and Wheal, *Stealing Fire.*

146   u/PabloAvocado, "Meditation vs Microdosing," r/microdosing, Reddit, May 3, 2017, https://www.reddit.com/r/microdosing/comments/68z5ji/meditation _vs_microdosing/.

147   "Getting into the Flow: Sexual Pleasure is a Kind of Trance," Northwestern University, EurekAlert!, October 31, 2016, https://www.eurekalert.org/pub _releases/2016-10/nu-git103116.php.

148   Jenny Wade, *Transcendent Sex: When Lovemaking Opens the Veil* (New York: Pocket Books, 2004).

149   Nicole Daedone, "TEDxSF—Nicole Daedone—Orgasm: The Cure for Hunger in the Western Woman," TEDx Talks, June 11, 2011, YouTube video, 15:07, https://www.youtube.com/watch?v=s9QVq0EM6g4&vl=en.

150   Nitasha Tiku, "My Life with the Thrill-Clit Cult," *Gawker* (blog), October 16, 2013, http://gawker.com/my-life-with-the-thrill-clit-cult-1445204953.

151   J. K. Ambler et al., "Consensual BDSM Facilitates Role-Specific Altered States of Consciousness: A Preliminary Study," *Psychology of Consciousness: Theory, Research, and Practice* 4, no. 1 (September 2016): 75-91, https://psycnet.apa.org /doi/10.1037/cns0000097.

152   Christopher Bergland, "Superfluidity and the Transcendent Ecstasy of Extreme Sports," *Psychology Today*, May 10, 2017, https://www.psychologytoday.com/blog /the-athletes-way/201705/ superfluidity-and-the-transcendent-ecstasy-extreme-sports.

153   Vincent Horn, "Meditation and Psychedelics," April 30, 2017, in *The Third Wave*, podcast, 1:18:47, https://thethirdwave.co/vince-horn/.

154   Dominic Barton and Gautam Kumra, "Leading in the 21st Century," *Mint*, December 4, 2013, https://www.livemint.com/Specials/JHQvjjJbYjmlsnImqy 600K/Leading-in-the-21st-Century.html.

155 Barton and Kumra, "Leading in the 21st Century"; Alison Griswold, "Nobody Likes Uber Anymore," *Quartz*, February 23, 2017, https://qz.com/917179/uber-is-racking-up-one-star-reviews-in-the-ios-app-store/.

156 Griswold, "Nobody Likes Uber Anymore."

157 Tony Schwartz, "How to Become a More Well-Rounded Leader," *Harvard Business Review*, July 21, 2017, https://hbr.org/2017/07/how-to-become-a-more-well-rounded-leader.

158 Taylor Pearson, *The End of Jobs: Money, Meaning and Freedom Without the 9-to-5* (Lioncrest Publishing, 2015).

159 Dave Logan, John King, and Halee Fischer-Wright, *Tribal Leadership: Leveraging Natural Groups to Build a Thriving Organization* (New York: Harper Business, 2008).

160 This is also called the "Dunbar's Number," popularized by British anthropologist Robin Dunbar, who found a correlation between primate brain size and average social group size.

161 Waldman, *A Really Good Day*.

162 Fadiman and Korb, "Microdosing," YouTube video.

163 Stephie Grob Plante, "LSD Microdoses Make People Feel Sharper, and Scientists Want to Know How," *The Verge* April 24, 2017, http://www.theverge.com/2017/4/24/15403644/microdosing-lsd-acid-productivity-benefits-brain-studies.

CPSIA information can be obtained
at www.ICGtesting.com
Printed in the USA
LVHW102314170123
737380LV00017B/315